INTERMITTENT FASTING 16/8

Table of Contents

Introduction

In the Intermittent Fasting program, you alternate eating and fasting periods. The fasting is to be considered a period of time in which you give your body a rest and a chance to cleanse itself. It's like a detox. Not eating allows the body to heal and put to use the nutrients that it received.

The fasting also helps to avoid sugar spikes and crashes, your levels of insulin (sugar) will remain more stable. This is a good thing because consequently hunger stabilizes.

During fasting time, the body is going to burn fat. Extra calorie intake turns to fat that get stored in the body, as a "provision". The fasting is for the body to use that "provision" and burn it.

The body tends to burn energy that is immediately available (food you just ate). Unless it has to, it doesn't burn the "provision".

During the eating window, make sure you always have healthy options available. It's harder to resist certain foods when you are hungry and the contrary is also true so it's easy to resist if you are not as hungry. If you always have healthy options available, you are less likely to become really hungry.

As you continue on your healthy eating plan, eventually you'll end the constant hunger and low energy attacks (cravings) that are so common when you are not mindful of your eating habits.

So the idea of intermittent fasting is to follow these healthy guidelines during the eating window and to allow your body to clean up during fasting.

The intermittent fasting program can help you lose weight if you are aware (and therefore if you are able to avoid) of certain misperceptions.

For example, just because you are fasting for a certain period of time, that doesn't mean that you can overeat during the eating window.

Also, if you want to lose weight and feel healthier, you need to choose some kind of physical activity that appeals to you. It doesn't have to be extreme but you should be moving your body at least 20 minutes almost every day.

There are so many activities for you to choose from and you could even pick a workout video on YouTube and follow it, if you don't have time to go to the gym. Or, you could run, ride a bike, go for a swim, do some aerobics or Pilates, play tennis. The options are endless.

If you are following the intermittent fasting diet but you are not losing weight it might be that you are drinking your calories and you are not counting those. Beverages are as important as food. Many people drink their calories through sugar dense, carbonated sodas which are filled with chemicals and sugar, although some are not aware of that.

If during the eating window you have pancakes for breakfast, cupcakes in the afternoon and pizza for dinner, it doesn't matter if you are fasting, you are not going to lose weight or feel better.

Also, if that is the kind of food that you eat on a regular basis, it will be much harder for you to fast because food that is rich in carbs, simple carbs – like baked products, make you want more of the same.

As for any other things in life, it takes a little while to adjust to a new habit. So at first you might even feel worse than before and feel like you are always hungry. That is because the body is getting rid of all the toxins and – if you don't give up immediately – you will adapt.

Before you start fasting, experiment putting long periods of time between your meals this will help in addition to reducing simple carbs and sugar and increasing protein and fiber (more fruits and vegetables). Start doing this for about 3 weeks before you begin the new program.

Chapter 1 16:8 intermittent fasting method

As is it in the name, this method involves two periods, a 16-hour fasting period and an 8-hour period of eating. It is advisable to keep your feeding periods constant to make the body it easy for your body to adapt and make it easy to follow. You cannot switch the feeding times around, as you want every day. Ghrelin, the hunger hormone, is released in according to your eating pattern. Constant changing of your eating pattern with mess with your hormones and leave you feeling hungry all the time.

It is a very sustainable and easy to keep on doing since you do not go long without food and can fit into your schedule effortlessly. This is also because part of the period when your fasting is at night, so the fasting period seems shorter. An example of the 16:8 schedule is if you eat at 10 pm, you will fast until 2 pm the following day.

It is true that your body will get used to being in a fasted state, but the journey to that point is not that easy, as you will be going against your body's food desires. These craving will be most powerful in the first two weeks but will greatly reduce after. So how do you deal with these cravings and keep on fasting?

1. Set clear goals that you want to achieve. What do you aim to accomplish with this fasting regiment? As it gets tougher, goals like wanting to get fit, health or burn some fat will not motivate you at all. If you do not have a clear reason for doing a fast, you are more likely to quit than someone who has specific goals. You should know what you want to achieve soon and in the long run. All these and more are the questions you should be asking yourself. Even after knowing what you want in those time periods, you should also ask yourself the reason for wanting those things and the effect of the objective to your life if it is achieved. This helps you to see things in a way that is more relevant to you. If you have the urge to eat that extra piece of cake, remember how in the end, if you achieve your goal, your life will change.

2. Make it a point to know why you are craving a certain food. Is it because of actual thirst and hunger because of boredom? Are you just

tired or stressed and looking for comfort in food? Try your best to distract yourself so that you do not end up eating during your fasting period. You should always give yourself-hope that you will make it through the craving period. It will pass, it always does.

3. Different things, in this book we will only talk about food, tempt us all at times. Removing temptation foods from your house will make it a lot easier to not be tempted to eat them.

4. If following recipes too tough at first, you can substitute them with shakes as you get used to it.

5. Organize your schedule. You may choose an eating window and discover that you do not have time to eat at that time. Do not set your eating window at a time you know it will be hard to go without food like if you eat when you are bored then don't set your eating period during the slowest part of the day. If you have, a meal with your family at a certain time then put your eating window at that time. Make wise choices when deciding your

feeding window. It always best to make it as easy as possible for you to follow.

6. Be your own support pillar. When you are starving, there is always this voice in your head that gives you many reasons why it is good to break your diet. It happens to us all when we are vulnerable. It is important for you to not listen to that voice. Even if you break the fast just once, you will eventually do it repeatedly. It is best to stay strong. If you give in, it happens to even the best of fasters, then do not use it as an excuse to stop fasting completely, keep on going because you only truly fail when you stop trying.

7. On top of personal support, also external support can help you. Make it a point to be around positive people who are on the same path as you. It will get hard and quitting will seem like the only option but if you have other people supporting you, it will keep you going. The more the better, you will be able to support each other, and you will all eventually reach your targets.

8. Stay hydrated. Dehydration sometimes may be interpreted as hunger by the body. Sometimes you might think that you are hungry while in actual sense you are just thirsty. Drink lots of water, black coffee, sparkling water, black tea or any other drink, which has zero calories.

9. Be patient. You may think of intermittent fasting as the magic bullet you can use to burn all your fat instantly but that is not possible. All good things take time, so does burning fat. You cannot workout and fast for two days and expect to have lost many pounds, do not get frustrated. You will only be able to see good results if you remain consistent through the process.

10. Give your body time to adapt to fasting. No living organism accepts change easily, your body will have to get used to the new way of life you have chosen and can react differently to fewer meals. Among the possible discomforts are headaches, hunger, and even body weakness. Better direction than speed, you might be moving slowly but in the right direction or you can be moving at supersonic speed in the wrong one. Do not give up.

One of the major factors that can help you succeed in intermittent fasting, which is overlooked by many, is sleep. The importance of sleep is not given enough weight by many books and articles on 16:8 intermittent fasting. Proper sleep can boost your overall fasting results by a large percentage. When you sleep, our bodies repair the damage, burn fat and replace cells. In sleep, both the quality and the quantity matter.

There are various ways of improving the quality of your sleep. First, get more sunlight. You "body clock" does not understand time the same way you do, it knows the time by light signals. Sunlight heavily influences it. Morning sunlight signals your glands and organs to wake up and make them produce hormones that should be used in the day. If you get a little sunlight in the day and on top of that, a lot of artificial light in the night, our circadian clock gets messed up. This malfunction can make your body produce hormones that can prevent you from sleeping. If you do not get enough quality sleep, there can be an increase in hormones such as insulin and hindrance to the production of hormones such as HGH causing no fat to be burnt at night.

You should also make it a point to avoid screens before bedtime. If you fall asleep watching TV or using your phone, it is best to keep away from them. Your body clock is not only affected by sunlight but also artificial light. These screens mostly produce blue light, which makes our body produce hormones that were meant to keep you awake and active. Falling asleep will be hard. Do not make it a habit of sleeping while using these devices. It is best to sleep in darkness. It is easier to sleep that way plus it can help you sleep better. Blackout your windows or put up heavy-duty curtains if there are annoying streetlights and other outside light sources that you cannot control.

There is a certain period in the night as you sleep that your body produces the best number of hormones required for fat burning and repair. It is best, if possible, to get into bed as once darkness falls. Healthy life, weight loss, and muscle building are just some of the many benefits of improving your sleeping habits. It may even do more than increasing the hours you spend in the gym.

Chapter 2 The Benefits of 16:8 Intermittent Fasting for Your Health

Intermittent fasting techniques, including the 16:8 method, are most commonly used to assist in weight loss by the general population. The method has been tried by thousands of people and also scientifically proven to be a helpful resource in reducing body fat and improving body composition. Weight loss is often considered the number one reason why people opt for a diet and program that utilizes intermittent fasting, in fact.

While a reduction in body fat is definitely one of the best advantages to be mentioned in terms of intermittent fasting, there are more advantages that people gain when they decide that they are going to follow this type of program – especially if they truly commit to it and can implement self-control that ensures they do not give in to cravings.

Intermittent fasting is known to assist in improving your body composition as well, as I mentioned earlier. Body composition refers to a series of features – this includes your body fat percentage and lean muscle mass primarily. A program that utilizes intermittent fasting, along with an appropriate diet plan, will bring down your body fat percentage, and push up your lean muscle mass at the same time.

It is also important to note the benefits that are associated with weight loss for people with an excessive amount of fat distributed throughout their body. Since overweight and obesity is linked to so many chronic diseases that can truly make your life dreadful, losing even small amounts of weight can drastically reduce your risk of these diseases. Additionally, if you have already been diagnosed with a disease associated with obesity, reduced body weight may improve the symptoms that you are experiencing and help you get the disease under control.

Take type 2 diabetes, for example. In one study, scientists describe that factors such as proinflammatory markers, cytokines, hormones, glycerol, and nonesterified fatty acids are all increased among those people who are obese. In turn, these factors all have factors that link them to insulin resistance. When insulin resistance develops, it can continue to progress into type 2 diabetes if the affected person does not implement appropriate preventative measures.

When you develop type 2 diabetes, you become predisposed to many additional risks and complications. In fact, type 2 diabetes can cause severe complications that may not only lead to disability but also become life-threatening. This disease can also affect all of the body's most important organs, including the heart, and can damage various tissues, such as nerves, throughout the body.

In addition to assisting in reducing body weight and bringing down the risks associated with obesity, intermittent fasting has many other benefits that are also worth mentioning.

Through intermittent fasting, cellular changes may occur in the body. This can lead to levels of human growth hormones rising by as much as 500%. This leads to a faster rate of fat burning, while also producing an increase in muscle mass.

It has also been found that intermittent fasting can help to remove waste that has built up in cells within the human body and can also assist in the repair process of cells that have been damaged. This means cells in the body become more efficient in performing their specialized functions.

One study also explains how recent findings from scientists suggest that intermittent fasting helps to improve brain health and may play a crucial role in helping medical experts better understand how diseases like Parkinson's disease and Alzheimer's disease can be prevented in the future.

Furthermore, following an intermittent fasting plan can also help to reduce levels of inflammation within the human body, as well as help to fight against oxidative stress. Both of these factors are known to contribute to numerous chronic diseases significantly and can causes certain molecules to become damaged, which can inhibit their functionality within the body.

In one study, scientists tested how intermittent fasting would work on the brain health and cardiovascular health among a group of laboratory rats. They found significant improvements in various tests used to determine the well-being of these two crucial hormones of the body. The scientists also associated these improvements among the tested laboratory rats with the reduction in oxidative stress that were observed. Additionally, the scientists also observed an improvement in the cellular stress resistance ratings in these rats. What this means is that an intermittent fasting diet can help to reduce the effect that stress has on the body, and help to fight against the existing oxidative damage, often also referred to as free radical damage, that has already occurred.

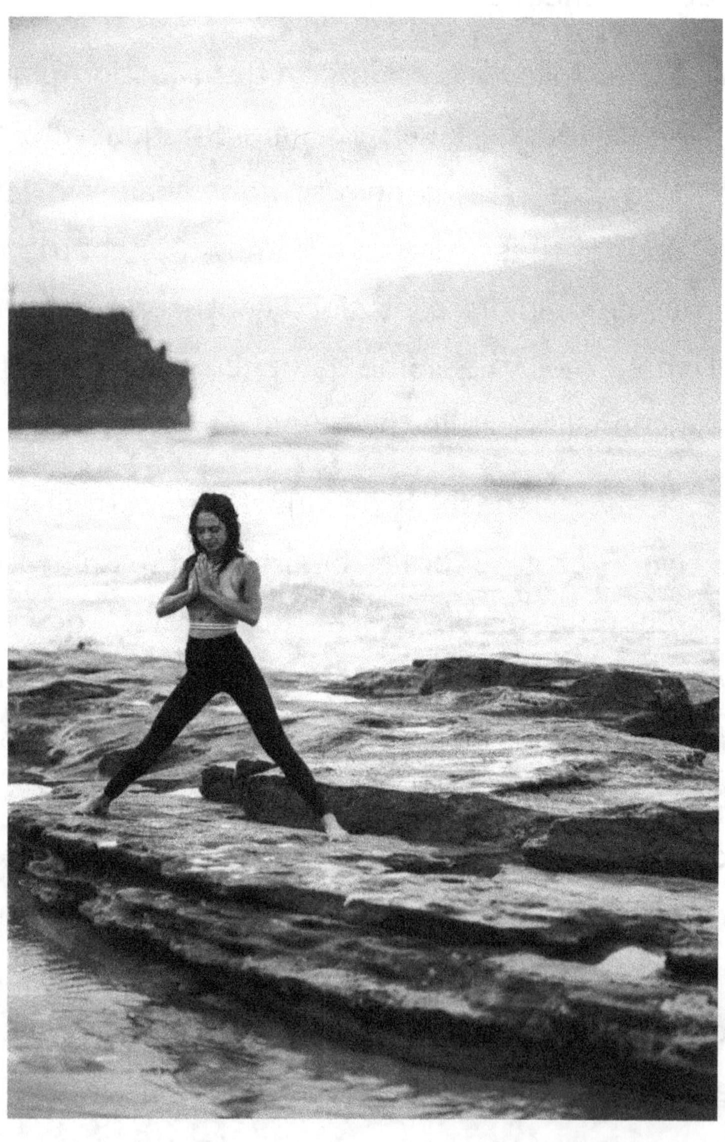

Chapter 3 Benefits of Dry Fasting

Research shows that going on a dry fast allows you to enjoy health benefits which include the following:

It removes toxins from the body.

Dry fasting helps cleanse your system. Research shows that going on a short intermittent 16/8 dry fast gives you the same results as a 3-day water fast. You get rid of the same level of toxic material and water weight from your body.

It decreases inflammation.

When you have an infection or even just a splinter on one of your fingers, your body goes into the defense mode. It goes through acute inflammation, a condition that increases the flow of blood (and body proteins and white blood cells with it) into the area at risk to fight infection and heal damaged tissue. The inflammation stops when the problem is resolved.

When the body has to deal with the constant or persistent presence of harmful elements, it experiences chronic inflammation. It stays on a continuous defense response.

Chronic inflammation can lead to damaged tissues and blood vessels, as well as to long-term health issues like cancer, type 2 diabetes, hypertension, and heart disease.

Your body secretes inflammation molecules or markers when your immune system has to battle infections. These markers and their effects on your body include the following:

The TNF-α molecule induces inflammation, fever, and loss of cells. It increases the risk of inflammatory bowel problems, psoriasis, Alzheimer's disease, and cancer.

High CRP levels indicate increased risk of cardiovascular problems, hypertension, and diabetes.

The IL-1b marker is closely identified with heart failure.

The IL-6 molecule aggravates autoimmune infections. It is also linked to increase chances of juvenile rheumatoid arthritis, diabetes, and malignant tumors in individuals who have breast cancer.

Research shows that going on dry fasts can help you significantly reduce the concentration of these inflammatory elements in the body.

It helps strengthen brain function.

Going on a dry fast enables the brain to release brain-derived neurotrophic factor or BDNF, a chemical that enhances brain functioning.

BDNF enhances learning and memory. It allows you to stock and retain information for future recall. It allows you to learn languages and new things, develop new skills, and engage in new activities even into old age.

BDNF strengthens the brain by creating new neurons. It also prevents brain cells from becoming weak and useless.

BDNF promotes the production of ketones, which keep the brain healthy. When the brain becomes over-stimulated, ketones have a significant calming effect that helps to lower anxiety and stress.

It keeps cholesterol levels on a healthy balance.

Going on a dry fast can boost HDL (the good cholesterol) and reduce LDL (the bad cholesterol). It can also bring down triglycerides and total cholesterol.

It helps in the regulation of blood sugar.

High blood sugar is linked to many health problems including kidney failure, nerve damage, heart problems, weak immune system, blindness, and erectile dysfunction.

Multiple studies indicate that people experience reduced blood sugar levels and higher sensitivity to insulin after going through a dry fast.

It prevents diabetes.

Going on a dry fast enables you to control your blood sugar levels As a result, you lower the risk of diabetes.

It prevents early osteoporosis.

Studies show that your body produces PTH or Parathyroid Hormone when you go through intermittent dry fasting. PTH spikes up calcium levels in your body. It also promotes healthy bone formation.

It helps you lose weight.

Going on a dry fast is a powerful technique for feeling lighter, burning fat, removing belly fat, and realizing your weight loss objectives.

It heals and strengthens the body through autophagy.

Abstaining from food and water or going on a dry fast is believed to be one of the most efficient ways to get the body to cleanse itself.

Autophagy is a natural process that the body uses to clean house. It is the body's natural and inherent recycling program.

Autophagy ("self-eating") is a process by which the body creates membranes that tracks down diseased, worn-out, or dead cells and "eats" them, using the subsequent molecules to produce new and well-functioning cell parts and sustain energy.

Autophagy makes the body efficient in getting rid of damaged cells, stopping cancerous tumors, and controlling diabetes, obesity, and other metabolic dysfunctions.

Autophagy controls inflammation. It enhances the body's innate ability to fight infection and diseases. It slows down the aging process.

The body normally gets rid of accumulated fats and toxic material through the skin, liver, kidneys, bowels, and urine. When you go on a dry fast, however, the body burns up waste material. A dry fast transform your body into an efficient waste-burning device that eliminates toxins. It initiates processes that enable the body to utilize everything on hand for fuel – at the cellular level.

It keeps you healthy and young.

Dry fasting stimulates and strengthens the immune system. It activates anti-inflammatory mechanisms. It cleanses the digestive tract and purifies blood. It helps cells regenerate.

All of these help you lose weight, boost energy, and acquire resilience and stamina. Your mind works faster and more clearly. Your body heals fast. You are able to fend off the early signs of aging.

As you can see from this long list of health benefits, dry fasting is the way to go if you want to become healthier and lead a longer, more energetic, and productive life.

Chapter 4 How to Start the Diet?

You've read quite a bit about intermittent fasting and beginning to think about how to start your diet. However, remember that this is a plan that does not restrict what you eat (although it does recommend steering clear of junk foods), but the times that you eat.

Yet, it can be overwhelming, making changes in the way you eat and probably in what you eat as well. You may be worried about the fasting part when you won't be eating. Maybe, you'll think that you can't get through your fasting period. Will you be hungry? Can you push through the times that you'll feel hungry? Will you be looking at the clock every five minutes until it's time to eat?

There is a much better way to start intermittent fasting, a calmer, confident way that you can prepare yourself to begin.

Instead of viewing it as something difficult, view it as something that is going to be beneficial for your health and well-being. Your goal is to lose weight, eat healthier, improve the functions of your body, and learn about it and consider it a self-experiment.

The best way to start is by breaking it down into small step-by-step procedures that will help you to succeed and guarantee you will achieve your goal. Analyze and observe what you discover and then come to your own conclusion and ask the question: Is intermittent fasting right for you?

Before You Get Started (Mindful Keto, n.d.)

Below are the steps to take before you start to implement your fasting plan:

Consult Your Health Professional

In many, if not all the chapters of this e-book, the same message has been given to you regarding consulting your healthcare professional. It is of the utmost importance that you see your physician before you begin intermittent fasting, for that matter, any diet plan you are attempting to begin.

This is especially true if you are taking any medication, especially for conditions such as type 2 diabetes, blood pressure, and any other ailments that can be affected by fasting. If you feel dizzy, nauseous, or cannot function, then you should stop the fast immediately and eat. Stop fasting if you feel sick.

Keep it Easy

Eat what you usually eat during your eating window. If possible, try to keep your meals low in carbohydrates and high in good fats and protein, fruits, and vegetables. Eat real, wholesome foods. Stay away from junk foods and processed luncheon meats. Eat fruits and vegetables. The goal, for now, is not getting the perfect mix of food combination to garner the best results. Your goal is to complete a fast. Starting out slowly will give your body (and your mind) to adjust to the newness of the way you will be eating and then fasting.

Don't allow the fears that may have held you back get in the way of you starting your fasting program. Remember, this is a learning process so that you can decide whether fasting is right for you.

Keep it Simple

For this fast, consume only carbonated or plain flat water, unsweetened tea, or black coffee. If you want a flavor for your water, squeeze some lemon juice or put in some sliced cucumber. You can also purchase unsweetened flavored water, but it's not necessary for this first time. Just remember not to add any cream or sugar to your coffee or tea.

What Time Will You Begin?

For the sake of simplicity, begin your fast at 8 pm. This is not something you have to follow, as intermittent fasting is flexible. You can choose any of the combinations of eating/fasting periods. The easiest one would be 16:8, where you eat for 8 hours and fast for 16 hours.

If you begin your fast at 7 pm, you will be able to eat again beginning at 12 noon the next day. If you have a conventional 9 am-5 pm job, this could possibly make the most sense because you will be breaking your fast at lunchtime. Remember that a large portion of the 16 hours in the fasting window, you'll be asleep. You'll be able to drink a morning coffee or tea and water until it's time to break your fast. .

Choose Which Days of the Week?

This is entirely up to you. Weekdays can make fasting easier because there is more structured with fewer variables. What you would want to do is look for the days where you would be surprised at how fast the time has flown by.

If you are going to adopt the 5:2 method, eating for five days a week normally and fast for two days, the choice is yours. You may choose Monday as a fast day in order to rid your body of the weekend toxins and then again on Thursday, so you can have the weekend as part of your eating period. However, it's entirely up to you and what fits your schedule and lifestyle.

Forgive Your Slip-Ups

You need to learn to forgive yourself if you slip up. If you do, pick up where you were or begin again from Day 1. Whatever is easiest, just do it and get back on track. Don't beat yourself up (we're all human) and whatever you do, don't give up and binge out.

What is Your Purpose?

This is when you question yourself and ask *why*? What is the purpose and what is the reason you want to intermittent fast? What do you want to derive from this experience?

Weight loss and maintenance – Fasting will increase HGH, the hormone that makes body fat that is stored more available to burn for energy, so you lose fat and norepinephrine and reduce insulin.

Relieve symptoms, relieve medication – Heart disease, diabetes, and reduced inflammation is prevented and are helped when you fast.

Promotes longevity, prevent serious disease– Studies have shown that you can be protected from Alzheimer's Disease and cancer when you fast, as well as help you to live longer.

Take Precautions

Pregnancy

If you're pregnant or lactating, intermittent fasting is not something you can do. A study examined the effects of Ramadan fasting (28 to 30 days and lasts from sun up to sunset each day) on the quality of breastmilk and discovered that it had deficiencies in important micronutrients like zinc, magnesium, and potassium. These are important nutrients that are necessary for babies and may put them at risk of being nutrient deficient.

Diabetes

If you're a diabetic, fasting is something that you need to be careful with due to insulin and blood sugar levels. Speak with your healthcare professional and if you do get the okay, monitor your blood glucose levels while fasting. If you are on insulin, it may need to change the dosage since fasting impacts on blood glucose levels.

Electrolyte imbalances

When you're fasting, keep in mind your electrolytes and fluid intake. Some people may avoid taking anything during their fast, but it's better to drink fluids to remain healthy and functioning. If you're working, highly active, and over the summer, it's good to monitor any imbalances that can arise.

Chapter 5 Combining Specific Diets and Intermittent Fasting

As we start looking into what we eat, it's important to discuss the possibility of "supercharging" your fast by adding a diet. Before we get into the different types of diets you can combine with the 16/8 method of intermittent fasting, it's important to make sure you understand the goals. We'll also discuss the benefits and risks and when to combine the two. Before you consider adding a diet to your fast, please make sure you talk to a doctor, especially if you have a medical condition you're concerned about.

Intermittent fasting isn't a diet. It doesn't require any changes to the type of food you eat, though that's recommended if you want to reap the most benefits. While most people will simply eat well-balanced, nutritious meals, you may want to add a diet if you have a very specific goal. If you are already dieting and you want to add intermittent fasting to your eating plan, then that's great! Just keep in mind that fasting will add some additional stress to your body, and it won't be compatible with some diets. Some example diets that don't work with intermittent fasting are very-low-calorie diets, diets that only focus on one or two food items, and any diet that is marketed as a cleanse.

Very low-calorie diets (like 800 calories a day) and fasting don't mix for some pretty obvious reasons. If you're not getting enough calories and you're not eating frequently, then you've created a dangerous recipe. Your body won't do well with such a restriction, and it's likely that you'll be malnourished and go into "starvation mode," where your body starts slowing down your metabolism. So, you won't see any results with this type of diet.

Diets that focus only on one food item or group will also backfire with a fasting diet. Fasting requires you to have enough energy from your food to make sure you're functioning well during your day, but if your food choice is only, say, cabbage soup, you're not going to get the right nutrients to power your day. You'll end up feeling weak, faint, or nauseous. It's also likely that remaining on such a diet will cause you to have some malnourishment, as there is no way you're getting enough nutrition from cabbage soup alone.

Finally, diets that claim to be "cleansing" diets won't really work with fasting. This is because most cleansing diets are liquid-based and don't really offer nutrition.

You will feel incredibly hungry on these cleanses while also fasting. Cleanses aren't necessary since your body can handle itself. So instead, choose diets that are nutritious, healthy, and will provide your body with enough energy to get through your fasting period.

There are two diets that do work well with intermittent fasting and have some scientific research to back it up. These two diets are the keto diet and some basic calorie restriction. Some people do more calorie restriction than the unplanned version that naturally comes with fasting but still eat more than 1,200 calories a day. Whichever way you choose, please proceed with caution. You don't want to end up in a state where you are shaking and have a foggy mind. Let's look at these two types of diets.

Keto

The keto diet can help people lose weight, but did you also know that it has been historically used to reduce epilepsy? The keto diet can also help with several diseases like diabetes, skin issues, heart disease, and cancer (Paoli et al., 2013). There is a lot of research to back up these claims. While most people today use the diet to lose weight, it's also a great option for people who are struggling with a variety of diseases. It uses food as medicine to help heal your body. For people who have epilepsy, eating very low-carb foods every day can help ease symptoms and even replace medications. Of course, please just don't throw your meds out. Talk to your doctor first.

So, the keto diet has a lot of positives, but why does it work? In the keto diet, you reduce your carbohydrates and increase your healthy fats and proteins. Your carbs are greatly reduced. It's not just a low-carb diet but a very-low-carb diet. Instead of eating carbs, you're eating more healthy fats. The whole purpose of the keto diet is to put your body in a state of ketosis. In this state, your body starts burning a lot of your stored fat instead of taking energy from carbs (that you're no longer eating). This may sound familiar since intermittent fasting does a very similar thing. It also puts your body into a state of using your stores of fat during the fasting period rather than using what you recently ate. Therefore the keto diet and intermittent fasting can work together so well.

Ketosis is a state where the body uses fat for energy. The body uses ketones to fuel itself instead of relying on glucose, which is what we get out of carbs and sugary foods. The science behind ketosis and reaching that state is beyond this book's purpose. So, to get to the point, to follow the keto diet, you need to reach the stage of ketosis. To reach this metabolic state, you must consume less than 50 grams of carbohydrates a day. That is not a lot at all. This is about 5% of your daily nutrition in comparison to our normal carb intake, which is well over 50% of our daily nutrition. So, it can be a little difficult to start the process of reducing carbs in such a drastic way.

Ketosis shouldn't be confused with ketoacidosis. Ketosis is healthy. Ketoacidosis is not. Ketoacidosis can affect someone with uncontrollable diabetes or uncontrollable alcohol consumption. It is the result of very high blood sugar levels that then turn your normal, benign blood into something that is highly acidic. Acid running through your veins is not healthy. If left untreated, ketoacidosis is deadly.

So, the keto diet's purpose is to get you into the state of ketosis. It's in this state that you'll burn your fat stores and lose weight. You'll also reap the other benefits of ketosis. Because you are losing your fat stores, you don't have to count your calories. You'll still eat large portions, just without the carbs. The absence of carbs means that you won't be converting it into stores of fat for later energy. You'll be replacing the carbs with higher amounts of healthy fats and proteins. This means you'll feel fuller longer and eating this way will suppress some of your appetite and cravings.

Combining fasting with the keto diet can help you shed more weight and reach ketosis faster than doing the keto diet alone. This is because fasting already primes your body to burn more fat instead of requiring carbs for an energy source. This is something closely connected to the keto diet.

Calorie Restriction

Calorie restriction is your typical diet. It's what most doctors and nutritionists recommend helping you lose weight. With calorie restriction, you are greatly reducing the number of calories you are eating each day. This results in weight loss because you simply are not eating as much as you used to.

To determine how many calories to reduce, you can use a calorie calculator online. You'll input information like your age, sex, height, and current weight. The calculator will give you information for the calories you need to eat to maintain your current weight and calories to eat to lose weight. All this calculation is just the beginning, though. You must do something with the information.

To do calorie restriction, you'll have to count your calories for every food item you eat. You can do this with apps that can calculate your calories based on food items. This is helpful for items that didn't come in a package. There isn't a "required" food to eat, but generally, you want to have a well-balanced diet when doing calorie restriction. This is because if you don't, your body may interpret your diet as starvation. The results of this will be some severe physiological responses.

The 16/8 method of intermittent fasting can result in unplanned calorie restriction, but you can up it a bit by doing it on purpose. Start by calculating the calories you need to eat to lose weight while also not being malnourished, and then plan your meals accordingly. Remember to keep your meals well balanced and record all the calories you eat.

Benefits and Risks

So, combining the keto and intermittent fasting could lead to better glucose levels, lower insulin levels, and better weight loss. Combining calorie restriction with intermittent fasting can result in weight loss, better physiological health, and better aging.

The risks associated with combining intermittent fasting and the keto diet or calorie restriction and the 16/8 method are like the risks already mentioned in chapter one. It's important to talk to your doctor or nutritionist before combining the fast with a diet. This will help you plan the appropriate steps and better understand the risks associated with combining.

Some people may find it difficult to start and maintain the keto diet. Since it's a restrictive diet, a lot of people's favorite foods may not fit into the diet. This can cause some people to struggle. A way to go about reducing this discomfort is to make the change slowly. Just like we do for intermittent fasting, take a couple of weeks to make your changes so that it's not such a jarring huge change. This may make it easier to follow the keto diet.

When first starting keto, a lot of people feel some physiological changes that aren't positive. This includes poor sleep, a feeling of fogginess, and digestive issues. It can also cause some difficulty with your energy levels, and this includes when you exercise. You'll need to be prepared for any of these feelings, and they'll pass after a couple of weeks while following keto.

There is an additional risk that you may lose some muscle when dieting with keto or doing calorie restriction. This is a risk that comes with any diet. Your body will start taking energy from your muscles instead of your fats if you're not getting enough protein or nutrients. To reduce this risk, make sure that you are eating enough and that it is well-balanced food. Don't just eat junk and expect your body to be okay with it. You'll lose more muscle like that.

With calorie restriction, there are risks like restricting your calories too much. If you do this while on a fast, your body will go into starvation mode, and you won't lose any weight. In fact, each time you eat, your body will start storing energy to prepare for the "starvation" period. Another risk is that you won't eat enough high-quality meals. This can lead to hunger during your fasting window. This isn't ideal, obviously. So, to combat this, make sure you eat well-balanced meals as part of your calorie restriction. It's important to get enough nutrition, so don't base all your food around one food group only.

When to Combine Them

If you're interested in following a specific diet while following your 16/8 fast, then there are a couple of ways you can combine them. First off, it's not recommended to start them both at the same time. Do you remember how we discussed making big goals and how they fail? Combining intermittent fasting with a diet right off the bat is a huge goal. Not only are you changing when you eat, but now you're also changing what you eat at the same time. That's a lot of change. It will cause your body a lot of stress, especially as you keep extending your fasting window. Instead, it's better to start either you diet first or your fast. Then later, you add the second part.

If you're going to start your diet first, follow your normal eating schedule. Change what you eat to fit your diet's requirements. If you're following the keto diet, this is a good way to start changing your metabolic state, which will also be enhanced by fasting at a later point. Remember that with the keto diet, you're going to have several weeks of discomfort as your body shifts into ketosis. This discomfort will pass eventually, so don't be alarmed. You'll notice things like changes in bowel movements, having different energy levels, and having mood swings. These symptoms won't pass very quickly, so take your time easing into the diet and getting past the symptoms.

Once you're well situated in the keto diet and you've been symptom-free for a while, you can start adding fasting to your diet. Again, ease into the fast and be prepared for your body's reaction to this change. If you are following the keto diet on your doctor's orders, please make sure you talk to them before adding the fasting component. You don't want to make too many changes to your metabolic levels without your doctor knowing if they gave you the green light for keto. If you're going at it alone and are already relatively healthy, then combine the two diets, and if you feel any severe discomfort, talk to your doctor.

If you're going to start with caloric restriction first, then again follow your normal eating times. Make sure that you are well versed in how many calories you can eat per day and what foods help you meet those goals. As you change your calorie intake, you may feel hungry more often and may experience feelings like fatigue and weakness. If the discomfort becomes severe, talk to your doctor. Once you've been following your calorie changes for a while and once you've reached a point where it feels comfortable, you can combine it with your fast. Here, you want to make sure that your fast doesn't result in further calorie restrictions. So, you want to be very consistent with what you're eating and make sure you are always counting calories. Your daily calorie limit should not change once you start your fast because you're already at a reduced calorie limit. If it does change, you're at risk for malnourishment and other side effects from the fast itself. It is very important that you keep a record of your calorie intake while you fast if you are following a calorie-restricted diet.

If you decide to try fasting before adding on diets, make sure you are taking the time to ease into the fast. You also want to make sure you're eating those well-balanced meals we keep talking about. This will help you transition easier into the fast. Once you've been following the 16/8 fast for a while, try incorporating your diet of choice. If you want to follow the keto diet, then make sure that you are cutting down on the carbs. This will push your body into ketosis. You may feel a lot of discomfort with this change, as your body will need to adapt to the new eating pattern you're following. If you decide to try calorie restriction, start by calculating how many calories you're currently eating in a day while fasting. Do this for a week. There's a chance that you're already eating fewer calories and already at your calorie goal for weight loss. So, it's important to check first. If you still need to cut calories, then do so carefully. You want to make sure that you still have enough food to keep you energized through your fast.

Throughout this entire process, keep journaling about your progress. This will help you keep on track, but also it will help you find areas that need improvement. Journaling is also a great way to keep track of foods, diets, or eating times that didn't work for you and why. This way, you won't do the same thing again. Now that we've talked about combining diets with the 16/8 method, let's look at what to eat while intermittent fasting.

Chapter 6 Nutrition

Intermittent fasting is very lenient as far as nutrition is concerned. By being lenient means, you are not restricted from eating anything in particular. You can eat pretty much anything within reasonable limits once in a while. It means if you have to attend a birthday party of a friend or any other celebration, then you wouldn't have to think a million times before having a piece of cake, or any other dessert.

You can enjoy a piece without carrying the burden of guilt upon yourself. However, this liberty comes with a caveat. You must eat it within reasonable limits. This liberty helps in keeping the temptations away. People who are tied under restrictions in eating often feel depressed and crushed. It leads to pessimism and negativity.

Remember, intermittent fasting is less about what you eat, and more about when you eat. As long as you are following the fasting hours, your body will be able to bear the once in a while indulgences.

Intermittent fasting limits the number of hours within which you can eat. It can mean a lot for people who have a habit of snacking frequently. Intermittent fasting schedule would limit the number of meals you can take, and hence, you will have to draw your whole nutrition from 2-3 meals within the 8-10 hours eating window.

Moving on from one meal to another can get difficult if you are not having balanced meals. If you are consuming too many refined carbs, then also, you might find it difficult to move on from one meal to another without feeling the food cravings and hunger pangs.

Therefore, it is very important that you have a very balanced meal.

Managing the Macronutrients

There are 3 main components of any meal

1. Fat
2. Protein
3. Carbohydrate

You must consume all these macronutrients in a balanced manner. Having a nutrient dense meal always helps in curbing hunger pangs for long, and suppressing the food cravings.

The ideal distribution of the macronutrients should be in the ratio given below:

Fat: 70-75%

Fat is dense, and the body takes a lot of time to process fats. This means that when you consume a fat-rich diet, it keeps you feeling full for longer, and prevents hunger pangs. The body takes much longer in processing the fats, and this also helps in preventing the insulin spike in your body. You can easily get a lot of calories even by eating fat in small quantities. When you have to consume a lot of calories in fewer meals, making fat the main component of your meal always helps.

However, you must ensure that you eat healthy fats. You can get healthy fats from animal meat, fish, nuts, seeds, and fruits. 1 gram of fat provides 9 calories. It is more than double the number of calories received from carbs of the same weight. This means you can get more calories by consuming fat in smaller quantities. You must include healthy fats in your diet to stay satiated.

Protein: 20-25%

Protein is essential for your muscles building. When your body is running on a low-carb diet, and you are doing a lot of exercises, there is a loss of muscle mass. The muscles are constantly breaking, and new ones are building. To help this process, you will need to consume a lot of protein. Therefore, protein should form the second biggest part of your meals. However, you should never consume protein in excess as that would again get broken as glucose.

You can get protein from lean meats, fish, nuts, dairy, egg white, and legumes. Try to have protein in moderate amounts to ensure that you get the required protein from your meals.

Carbohydrate: 5-10%

Carbohydrate should constitute the smallest part of your meal. You must not consume refined carbs as they get processed very quickly, and increase the blood sugar levels. However, once the body processes the refined carbs, you would start feeling hungry again. Consumption of refined carbs would lead to food cravings and hunger pangs.

You must consume complex carbohydrates like whole grains that take a lot of time to get processed, and give your gut a lot of fiber in the end. This not only helps in keeping your blood sugar levels low, but is also very good for your gut ecosystem. There are several important trace minerals that are only found in whole grains, and that's why they are so important.

Green leafy vegetables are the second most important source of carbohydrates that you must consume. Green leafy vegetables do not only have a lot of fiber, but also vitamins and minerals in huge quantities. They help you with a lot of antioxidants, phytonutrients, and flavonoids that are helpful in fighting chronic inflammations. You must consume at least 7-8 cups of green leafy vegetables every day for a healthy body.

There are several benefits of consuming green leafy vegetables in large quantities. First, they are very low in calories, and hence you can consume them in any quantity you like without worrying about the calories consumed. Second, the green leafy vegetables provide a gel-like fiber to your body that helps your gut a lot. It helps in keeping your digestive system clean. You wouldn't face problems like constipation and other such issues. Third, green leafy vegetables can be consumed in large quantities, and hence they help you in feeling fuller for longer.

You can eat them as salads, or even make a smoothie as per your liking. However, it is always advisable to avoid starchy vegetables in large quantities, as they just add calories to your system and raise your blood sugar levels.

Things to Avoid

Fruit Juices: It is never advisable to have fruit juices. Fresh or packed, fruit juices are not good for your body. They raise your blood sugar levels instantly without adding fiber to your system. Drinking juice is like adding empty calories to your system.

Soda and other caloric beverages: Like juices, they also add empty calories to your system. In addition, they are even worse for your body as they are prepared from refined sugar. You will start feeling cravings to have more soon after you have some.

Refined flours: Refined flours and the products made from them are bad for your health. These flours do not have the original fiber content, and are very easy to process. This means that after consuming refined flours, you will again start feeling hungry very soon. They are bad for your digestive system and raise your blood sugar levels very fast.

Sugar: Sugar in any form should be avoided. You must buy everything after checking the label. If it has sugar, maple syrup, fructose, or any other such thing at the top of the ingredient list, it must be avoided. Such things will make your fasting routine very difficult as you will have food cravings and frequent hunger pangs.

Processed Food: Processed food items are bad for your health. To increase the shelf life of processed food items, a lot of sugar is added to them. In place of healthy fats, trans fats and hydrogenated fats are used. All these things are very bad for your health, hence, you must avoid them at all costs.

Trans Fats: Trans fats are bad, and although most processed food items don't have trans fat listed as an ingredient, or its value is given as zero, it is not the whole truth. The best way is to avoid highly processed food items, especially the ones with a lot of added preservatives

Chapter 7 Exercise

Exercising is important as it helps in burning fat faster. It is also important for building healthier muscles. All those people who have been objecting exercise in a fasted state only explain one side of the story.

There are a few things on which everyone agrees:

1. Exercises help in burning fat
2. They help in keeping the body fit
3. They also help in uplifting your mood and bringing positivity

Now, some experts believe that when you exercise in the fasted state, your body feels the energy crunch, and tries to break muscles as calories. This will happen because, after carbs end, the muscles are the easiest form of energy. The muscles are made of protein, and protein can also be broken down easily. However, it isn't that simple.

Although it is correct that some muscle loss takes place while you are doing exercise, it is wrong to assume that it happens because your body is trying to produce energy from them. Some amount of loss of muscle mass would take place even after you have had a high dose of glucose drink. This happens because the muscles are continuously getting damaged during exercise, and they break apart to give way to stronger ones.

Once your body has exhausted the glucose and glycogen reserves, it starts burning the fat reserves for energy. The fat is a more reliable and long-lasting source of energy, and it can fulfill all the energy needs of the body without causing any harm. To think that the body would think or behave otherwise is irrational.

The HGH Story

Our body produces an amazing hormone by the name of Human Growth Hormone. The production of this hormone is very high during our growing years as it helps in the building of bones, muscles, and every other part of our body. The production of this hormone is at its peak when we reach puberty, as we start growing at an immense rate all of a sudden. However, as soon as we cross our teens, the production of this hormone slows down as our body realizes that it has stopped growing at a fast pace.

However, our body never stops producing HGH completely. It keeps producing this hormone is short spurts. It is still a hormone that helps in growth and repair. So whenever you are in trauma or great pain, the production of this hormone increases.

Under normal circumstances, there are some specific conditions under which the production of HGH increases:

- When you are sleeping
- When the production of 'ghrelin', the hunger hormone is high in your gut
- When the insulin levels are the lowest in your gut

This increases the production of HGH in your body. This hormone can do some wonderful things. Among others, some important things are:

✓ It improves your stamina

✓ It accelerates fat burning

✓ It prevents loss of muscle mass

✓ It helps in the building new muscles

This means that when you do high-intensity exercise in the fasted state, the HGH in your blood would help in burning fat faster, and would also support building new muscles.

Therefore, you can exercise in the fasted state without having to worry a lot. The only thing you need to remember is that always increase your exercise timings slowly. Never start with bigger sets. Always build up your routine in stages.

HIIT

High-Intensity Interval Training is very helpful in burning fat, as you get to create huge energy demands that are to be met by burning fat. However, you must remember that HIIT puts a lot of pressure on your body, and hence, you must give your body the due rest after exercise.

HIIT should always be carried out on alternate days, so that the body gets proper rest and recovery time. On the alternate days when you are not doing HIIT, you can do light exercises like walking, jogging, swimming, yoga, and aerobic exercises.

Some Golden Rules to Safely Exercise While Fasting

Do HIIT Near the End of Your Fasting Schedule

If you keep your exercise routine close to the time of your ending the fast, you can get calories very soon. This is a good way to put a stop to all doubts of muscle loss. A protein rich diet at the end of your HIIT will help in removing all fears of muscle loss. It would also provide you the required energy.

Always Remain Hydrated

Dehydration can be more dangerous than the calorie deficit. You must always drink plenty of fluids to remain hydrated. Fasting only stops you from consuming calories. It has nothing against remaining hydrated. It is important for flushing out toxins and running the body smoothly.

Smaller Sets for Shorter Duration

The purpose of HIIT is to create sudden energy demands. If you stretch HIIT for too long, it can cause problems like muscle cramps. You must do small sets and keep taking breaks.

Always Listen to Your Body

Your fight must be against the fat and other physical ailments, but it isn't against your body. You must always listen to your body and pay heed to its demands. If you ever feel that the routine is getting overtaxing, you should take a break.

Chapter 8 Challenges of Intermittent Fasting

Intermittent fasting is a simple and effective weight loss plan, and it is safe for almost anyone to try. Fasting encourages healthy eating and increases your understanding of your body and the reasons for your hunger.

Many people have no issues transitioning to this new diet. For some people, though, there may be a few mild side effects that are noticed during the first few weeks of fasting. As soon as your body adapts, these should go away.

You may find that you feel uncomfortably full after eating, especially after your first large meal after a fast. Digesting a big meal can put stress on the body. If your schedule is such that you eat your biggest meal of the day at night, it may have a negative impact on your sleep as well. It is usually a good idea to keep this first meal after a fast, fairly moderate and healthy. If you experience trouble with overeating and end up feeling too full, try planning your meals in advance.

You may begin to obsess over what and when you will eat next. Some people will think about food obsessively when they first start to fast and end up watching the clock constantly. Overthinking about food should go away as your eating schedule becomes more natural to you. It might take about two weeks to adjust to your new plan and to stop thinking about the details so much. It is best to keep an eye on this symptom if it occurs so that the obsession does not lead to an eating disorder.

Hunger and food cravings. Fasting can make hunger more intense. However, your body should get used to this side effect over time. In the beginning, you may find that food is all you think about. You may crave sugar from time to time as your body is looking for a quick energy source. It will take a bit of willpower and some of the strategies mentioned above to get past some of the hunger.

Your workouts at the gym may be impacted. Some people do find it difficult to perform at the same physical level on an empty stomach. If this is the case for you, it might take some additional planning on your end to avoid working out near the end of a fasting cycle. When you work out, you lose a lot of water and sodium from your body through sweat. Rehydration following exercise will be an important step in your routine.

Heartburn – Your stomach produces acid to help with digestion. Intermittent fasting impacts the production of stomach acid, which in turn can lead to heartburn. Heartburn may be worse if you're eating window is later in the day. The good news is that this symptom usually goes away after a few weeks. In the meantime, it might be best to avoid eating foods that will make your heartburn worse. This includes heavily processed foods, some dairy, spicy foods, and foods that are high in acidities such as chocolate, coffee, onions, and garlic.

Headaches or dizziness– Some people experience headaches when they first begin on an intermittent fasting plan. Headaches are usually mild but may be reoccurring for the first few weeks of your transition. Dehydration will make headaches worse, so make sure you are drinking plenty of water during your fasts. You might also try adding salt to your water to make sure your electrolytes are staying in balance. See your doctor if your headaches continue for more than two weeks.

Diarrhea or constipation – The drop in insulin levels that are associated with intermittent fasting can sometimes signal the body to get rid of excess water. The result of this may be episodes of diarrhea. In addition, eating less food may also result in less movement of the bowels. Fasting can slow down the digestive system, which may cause constipation. For both of these conditions, drinking lots of water will help. Be patient as your digestive system stabilizes and becomes accustomed to your new way of eating.

Low energy or brain fog – When you first start on your intermittent fasting plan, you may feel sluggish, lethargic, or even weak at times. Keep in mind that on this plan, you are running on less fuel than you are used to. Feeling a bit low in energy is quite normal. Your energy levels may fluctuate quite a bit as you get started with the plan, but should even out after a few weeks. You may also experience some minor difficulties in concentrating, which is sometimes referred to as "brain fog."

Hormonal changes. Intermittent fasting affects hormone levels and functioning for women in particular.

Sleep Disturbances. Your sleep patterns and quality of sleep might be affected by this change in your lifestyle. You may find that both hunger pains and fluctuations in hormones might keep you awake at night. Your body tends to produce more adrenaline in response to a fast, as your metabolic rate receives a boost. This process can end up giving you energy at times when you would rather be sleeping or can make you feel a bit jittery.

Irritability – changing your eating habits may affect your mood. Some people get cranky or irritable when their blood sugar levels drop. Expect some minor changes in your mood or some mood swings as you get started.

Bad breath – A few people experience something called "keto breath" when fasting. The ketones that our body produces when in a fasted state are the cause of this nuisance. This side effect is more common for longer, extended fasts, and again, tends to go away with time.

Pay attention to any new or unusual symptoms that you experience during your fast, especially if you have never tried fasting before. If you do experience some side effects, do not give up on fasting too soon! You are putting your body through a change, and it needs time to adapt. If you experience dizziness, nausea, headaches, digestive issues, or low energy, it could be that you are not drinking enough water throughout the day. Having said that, do not ignore symptoms if they persist or become worse. If you feel unwell for more than a few weeks, take a break from fasting if you suspect that might be the cause. Make an appointment with your doctor to discuss whether fasting is the right lifestyle choice for you.

If you have any concerns about intermittent fasting, it is best to consult with your doctor ahead of time, especially if you are taking any medications that may be impacted by a change to your eating schedule.

Those with a history of an eating disorder or who are at risk of developing one should not fast. Risk factors include having a family member with an eating disorder, having a mood disorder, impulse control issues, or those who struggle with perfectionism. Fasting may increase your risk of developing anorexia or bulimia. Individuals who are underweight should not try intermittent fasting.

Additionally, children under the age of 18 should also refrain from fasting. Children require healthy, consistent meals while they are still growing and maturing. Children who are overweight should first remove all junk, processed foods, and foods that are high in sugar and fat from their diet. Adding regular exercise to the routine of an overweight child is also recommended for weight loss.

What to Eat and Drink While Fasting

During your fasting window, you should completely refrain from eating any food unless you are following the 5:2 method or modified alternate-day fasting. All food contains calories, and consuming calories elicits your body to start the digestive processes. Once you eat anything, you break your fast.

When fasting, it is vital that you drink more water than you normally would. A large amount of water that you normally take in comes from the foods that you eat, like fruits and vegetables. If you are not eating these water-dense foods, you need to make up for it by drinking more throughout the day. It is recommended that women drink at least 2.4 liters, or 11 cups of water a day. For men, 15 cups are the recommended number. As a loose rule, you should aim to drink about half of your body weight in ounces each day. For example, if you weigh 160 pounds, you should try to drink about 80 ounces of water per day.

Drinking plenty of fluids will help keep hunger pains at bay, which might make it easier for you to stick with your intermittent fasting plan. Water is good for you in other ways as well, it helps keep your joints lubricated, and your digestive system regulated. Water flushes our body of waste and helps maintain optimal body temperature. Drinking water helps release toxins from the body. It flushes them out and can be preventing headaches and muscle cramps. Water also helps burn fat faster, by extracting available nutrients from your body.

If drinking water on its own gets boring, think about adding natural flavor to it that does not contain any calories or sugar. Squeeze lemon, lime, mint, or cucumber into your water if you are craving something new. Before long, if you keep your water intake up and your calories down, your body will begin to crave water instead of food. You can also drink carbonated water, as long as there is no added sugar. Read labels carefully if you purchase carbonated water, to make sure there are no hidden ingredients in it.

Besides water, there are a few other calories-options that you can drink while you fast. It is okay to have unsweetened tea or black coffee. Consuming coffee without cream, milk, or sugar may help accelerate your metabolism, which helps promote weight loss, as well as reduce appetite. Use caution when drinking coffee, though. Too much caffeine may make you feel jittery or anxious, especially on an empty stomach. Caffeine can also impact the quality of sleep, sometimes leading to sleep disturbances and symptoms of insomnia. No more than 1-2 cups of coffee a day are recommended. If you would like to increase your coffee intake beyond this, try switching to decaf.

It is also fine to chew sugar-free gum while fasting, although there are mixed reports on whether this causes people to feel more or less hungry. It is best to stay away from sodas, even if they claim to be sugar-free, as well as artificially flavored drinks. These drinks are generally loaded with artificial sweeteners. Consuming them may lead to sugar cravings, and over time, may increase your insulin resistance.

Some experts suggest drinking diluted apple cider vinegar as a method of encouraging weight loss. Diluted in about 8 ounces of water, apple cider vinegar will not break your fast, and also offers a number of health benefits. It has been proven to be a positive influence on your metabolic system and may help to reduce levels of bad cholesterol.

Chapter 9 Mistakes to avoid committing

Sticking to an intermittent fasting approach will let you experience tremendous benefits, among which are better digestion, significant weight loss, minimal sugar cravings, better sleep, and improved mental clarity. However, your journey towards attaining your desired results will most likely be accompanied with some errors. While you can't perfect intermittent fasting for the entire period you are planning to do it, take note that there are some mistakes committed by other practitioners of this eating pattern that you can simply avoid.

Mistake #1 – Changing your eating habits drastically

If you are one of those whose normal eating habits include eating every three to four hours or so then shrinking the time you need to eat within just an 8-hour period all of a sudden can lead to certain issues, like extreme hunger and frustration.

A lot of people make the mistake of adding drastic changes into their lifestyle and eating patterns all of a sudden by trying to stick to a long fasting period.

You should avoid this mistake as much as possible if you want to succeed in IF.

Always remember that you might need around 10-14 days to finally adjust and prevent yourself from feeling extreme hunger during your fasting period. Avoid making the change in your eating habits all of a sudden. What you have to do, instead, is to stretch the amount of time in between your meals in a gradual manner (for instance, until you reach an eating window of 12 hours).

You should then move into an eating window of 10 hours. After that, reduce that window even further but only by small increments. Do this until you reached your target eating window.

Mistake #2 – Consuming the wrong liquids

Some people drink tea, black coffee, or water so they can go through their fasting period with the least amount of discomfort.

The problem is that if you can't tolerate black coffee then you may be tempted to add some sugar or milk without thinking about whether or not this will break your fast. Prior to adding anything to your drink, find out if it will affect your desired results first. If possible, do not let coconut oil and butter get near your coffee.

You should also stay away from liquids filled with protein, like bone broth. It is because these liquids have the ability to stop autophagy, which refers to a cellular process capable of breaking down and recycling damaged molecules. This is something that you may want to achieve when you are on your fasting period.

It is also advisable to stay away from diet sodas. You need to avoid anything, which is sweetened heavily, even those advertised as free of calories. Remember that even zero-calorie sweeteners can negatively affect your insulin level, which might also stimulate your appetite and cause cravings. To prevent taking in wrong liquids, keep track of your hydration and the specific drinks you take in.

This is a huge help in making yourself accountable and motivating yourself to stick to black coffee, plain tea, and water during the fasting period. Once you get used to drinking the right liquids, make sure that you do not forget to hydrate yourself, especially during the fasted state.

Note that while the IF regiment refrains you from eating foods during your fasting period, it is necessary for water or other healthy liquids to be close to you. It is mainly because this eating pattern might cause you to miss out on the kind of hydration often provided by healthy fruits and vegetables.

You do not want to suffer from dehydration as it has several side effects, like muscle cramps, hunger pangs, and headaches. With that in mind, ensure that you sip enough water and other allowed liquids all throughout the day regardless if you are in your eating or fasting window.

Mistake #3 – Leading a sedentary lifestyle

Working out when you are sticking to the intermittent fasting approach might seem like a new endeavor for you, especially if you are used to eating a pre-workout snack. However, this should not be a reason why you should lead a sedentary lifestyle during your fasted state. Note that even if you are fasting, you can't still lose weight if you do not pair it with proper exercise.

The good news is that your body actually stores plenty of energy in your body fat. This is what your body will use in case there is no food. With that in mind, it is possible for you to retain your usual exercise routines even when you have changed your eating pattern. If the entire experience is really new then you may want to try out low-impact exercises, like walking.

In case you decide to fast overnight and work out during the morning then it is advisable to consume a meal rich in protein after it. It is helpful in increasing your body's muscle-building rate. One thing to remember before pairing IF with your regular workout, though, is that just like other exercise or diet plans, you have to consult your doctor first. However, in general, pairing your regular exercises with IF is safe.

Mistake #4 – Sticking to the wrong intermittent fasting plan or approach

Note that for IF to produce favorable results, you need to pick the right plan – one that perfectly fits your lifestyle, current condition, and personality. Avoid making yourself miserable by trying to stick to a pattern, which is not compatible with your own lifestyle. If you know that you are a night owl, for instance, then avoid starting your fasting sessions every 6 pm.

In case you are someone who goes to the gym every day and do not want to sacrifice your daily workout then avoid picking an IF plan/method, which has severe calorie restrictions for several days every week. Consider your lifestyle and personality and find out which among the IF methods will work for you. By choosing the most suitable fasting method, it will be easier for you to stick to the new habit.

Mistake #5 – Beating yourself up in case you eat beyond your eating window

Do not feel too guilty if you slip up from the pattern sometimes. Avoid beating yourself up when you grab a food even if you are no longer in your eating window. Note that you need to listen to the cues sent by your body. If you feel real hunger then there is no reason to deprive yourself of what you need.

Remember that addressing your hunger is actually okay when doing intermittent fasting. Just make sure that you do not do it all the time. Also, one thing that you have to remind yourself on a constant basis is that if you deny your body's hunger cues then your relationship with food will become unhealthy.

Do not be too hard on yourself and allow it to break from the fast in case you truly feel hungry during your supposed-to-be fasting state. Keep in mind that the idea behind intermittent fasting is not to starve yourself. With that in mind, it is crucial to still provide yourself with the right nourishment, especially if you are starting to experience negative symptoms.

Mistake #6 – Restricting calories too much when the eating window comes

One problem experienced by those who just started following intermittent fasting is that the whole eating pattern causes them to continue restricting their calories even after breaking their fast. You do not have to be too strict and rigid by excessively restricting your calorie intake. Note that intermittent fasting also requires you to hear what your body is telling you. Listen to it and eat until you experience fullness.

The good news is that the human body is actually an incredible machine but you also have to let it to do its job correctly. In that case, you can expect it to release hormones that will let you know whether you are already full. You just have to watch out for the 1 it releases that signify fullness.

Avoid restricting your calorie intake too much during the time when you are supposed to eat. It is because doing so might only lead to under-eating, causing several unwanted body changes and long-term consequences.

Mistake #7 – Pushing yourself too hard

This is a mistake often committed by those who wish to try extending their fast for as long as possible even if it means forcing themselves. Some even go to the extent of fasting for more than 48 hours even if they already experience too much discomfort. You should determine whether the extended/prolonged fast works for you before trying it out first.

Keep in mind that you can't expect the process of extending your fast to supercharge IF and produce more incredible benefits. If you force yourself to fast for an extremely long period even to the point of extreme discomfort then consider seeking the help of a counselor whose specialty is on eating disorders. The foods you regularly eat should not cause regret and remorse, so seeking the help of a professional can be beneficial.

Also, take note that your poor relationship with food can produce even bigger problems in the future. This is why talking to a counselor is really advisable so you can figure out whether you already have an eating disorder or if your relationship with food is still healthy.

Mistake #8 – Obsessing over eating windows and schedules

One great benefit of intermittent fasting is that it teaches you to be fully in tune with your own body signals. It allows you to understand real hunger, which is something that happens every 16 to 24 hours instead of the every 4 hours that a lot of people believe. With that in mind, you do not have to obsess too much over your eating windows and schedules.

You have to make sure that your body dictates the perfect time for you to eat, instead of the clock. Focusing on time periods too much might cause you to count the hours left until your next meal. This will prevent you from learning and fully understanding the signals sent to you by your own body.

For instance, if you decide to skip breakfast then you are basically extending your fasting overnight to around 16 hours. Your focus should not be on the schedule or the time period. This means that in case you decide to skip breakfast, then you also have the option of breaking the fast once you feel hungry, although it is advisable to do this only occasionally.

Mistake #9 – Trying to do numerous things at once

You may be forcing yourself to do a lot of things while trying to practice the intermittent fasting approach. Some of the things you might do are over-training, dry fasting, and under-eating. Also, remember that if you are someone with poor eating habits and who lacks workout in the past and want to try intermittent fasting for better health then avoid biting more than what you can actually chew. This is important, especially if you are still a beginner.

Allow yourself to ease gradually into training and fasting. Also, avoid training 5 times weekly, fasting daily, and extremely restricting your calorie intake after fasting. It is because this might only trigger serious consequences in the future. One more thing to remind yourself is that your body survives with a bit of physical stress from time to time. However, you should try avoiding too much stress as this might produce more chronic issues.

Mistake #10 – Choosing the wrong foods

A lot of intermittent fasting followers also make the mistake of choosing the wrong foods. In fact, many of those who tried it think that it is a magic pill capable of solving their weight and health problems. While it is true that IF is an effective tool for those who want to have full control over their health and weight, it is still possible to cancel out its benefits if you eat the wrong foods, specifically processed and sugary ones, during your eating window.

Keep in mind that since you are fasting, it is more essential to give your body the right nourishment through whole and nutrient-dense foods. Being in the fasted state also encourages your body to break down any damaged parts then use these to produce energy. This is helpful in healing and cleansing your body. This also results to in body becoming more and more sensitive to all the foods you take in. Such sensitivity is beneficial if you take in foods rich in nutrients.

However, it will not do you any good if the foods you consume do not nourish your body. If that is the case, you will experience extreme hunger most of the time since your body will start to crave for nutrients. With that in mind, focus on consuming highly nutritious foods when it is already time to eat. Do not just focus on cutting calories. Your goal is to ensure that your body still receives sufficient amount of nutritious foods to ensure that your organs and your brain will continue to function well.

Intermittent Fasting myths

Intermittent fasting is one of the most rewarding eating patterns and lifestyle you can try. However, before starting your journey towards enjoying its numerous benefits, it is crucial to study the facts and myths behind it. This chapter will debunk some of the most famous intermittent fasting myths and offer truthful information about how this eating pattern really works.

Myth #1 – Intermittent fasting guarantees significant weight loss

Contrary to what most people believe, IF can't be expected to result in significant weight loss all the time. This is especially true if you are doing this approach the wrong way. Note that regardless of the length of your fast, you can't still expect to achieve the results you want as far as weight loss is concerned if you constantly include burgers, candies, pizzas, and other unhealthy foods during your eating period. You still need to pair IF with regular exercises and a healthy diet. You can't treat each eating period as a cheat day.

Myth #2 – Intermittent fasting leads to muscle loss

No, your muscles will not shrivel up and break down during your fasted state. Keep in mind that the human body stores two forms of energy, namely fat and sugar. This means that your body will only be using these two forms of stored energy.

Protein, which is a major component of your muscles, will not be used by your body to produce energy when you are fasting. What happens, instead, is that your body will make use of sugar as the primary source of fuel during the first 1-2 days without food.

After that, your body will begin opening up and accessing stored fats as a source of energy. This means that it will start breaking down the stored fats in your body to create fuel once your stored sugar depletes. Each person has around 50,000 to 100,000 calories of fat on average stored in his body, which is equal to almost one month's worth of available stored fats.

If you intend to fast, therefore, then you do not have to worry about your muscles breaking down since it is your stored fat and sugar that your body will use as fuel.

Myth #3 – Intermittent fasting can slow down your metabolism

You do not have to worry about intermittent fasting negatively affecting your metabolic rate. It is because the entire eating pattern will not slow down your metabolism. Keep in mind that IF does not involve excessive calorie restrictions. What it does is to restrict the time you consume calories.

A few more hours spent waiting to take your first meal does not have a major effect on your metabolic rate.

However, you should avoid under-eating during your eating period as this practice is the one that might send your metabolism downhill.

Myth #4 – Intermittent fasting can lead to poor brain performance

Glucose is your brain's main source of fuel. With that in mind, it is no longer surprising to see those who are planning to try IF worrying about being unable to give their brain a consistent supply of glucose. The truth, however, is that IF will not negatively affect the performance of your brain.

Keep in mind that your body is still capable of using stored fuel from your body to produce glucose. This means that even if you follow low-carb intermittent fasting approach, it is still possible for your brain to get a good supply of fuel through ketone bodies that break down fat.

Intermittent fasting can even lead to better mental performance, focus, and clarity. It is mainly because fasting can stimulate epinephrine and norepinephrine production. If you get into the fasting mode, your body will cause a minor stress response, which releases adrenaline. This breaks down the fats stored in your body as fuel, thereby providing you with the focus and energy you need.

Furthermore, fasting can lead to the production of BDNF (brain-derived neurotropic factor). This can help your existing neurons survive, stimulate the growth of new neurons, and improve your learning and thinking ability and your memory. It also helps lessen your risk of suffering from depression and Alzheimer's disease.

Chapter 10 Myths About Intermittent Fasting

There are many myths out there about Intermittent Fasting. the common myths are as follows;

MYTH: Your body will definitely enter in starvation mode.

TRUTH: Your body will not definitely enter in starvation mode through Intermittent Fasting. Skipping meals or adjusting to longer periods between meals where you don't eat is not going to make you starve. It's going to help your body remember how to absorb nutrients. It's going to help you thrive instead.

MYTH: You'll lose muscle in this endeavor.

TRUTH: This myth goes along the same lines as the first one, above. Just like your body won't enter the starvation mode (unless something goes very, very wrong or you're trying to do too much); your body won't lose muscle through IF. The only reason why intermittent fasting would cause muscle loss would be if it was causing you to starve, but once again, the first myth addresses this falsity, making this myth false as well.

MYTH: You'll almost assuredly overeat during eating windows, and that's not healthy at all.

TRUTH: While some people will have the instinct to overeat during eating windows, not everyone will overeat. Even those who do at the start will realize how to move forward without this overeating instinct in the future. Your body will urge you to overeat because, at the start, it won't realize what you're doing to it, but as long as you keep portion sizes largely the same and don't gorge on snacks, your body will adjust and so will your appetite.

MYTH: Your metabolism will slow down dangerously.

TRUTH: Your metabolism won't slow down just because you're eating less often. People who think this myth is true, only assume that restricted caloric intake will make one's metabolism slow down over time, but these individuals forget that IF isn't necessarily about cutting down calories overall. It's actually about cutting down the times during which one consumes calories. There needn't be any caloric restriction whatsoever! It just depends on the practitioner and what he or she decides to do with dieting in addition to IF.

MYTH: You'll only gain weight if you try skipping meals.

TRUTH: This myth is based on the same logic that drives the myth about overeating. If you gorge yourself during your eating windows, you'll surely gain weight, but hardly anyone will continuously gorge with IF. Anyone who tries will realize how unsuccessful it is, so he or she will not continuously gorge in response. Anyone who doesn't realize his or her efforts with eating are unsuccessful will soon realize that something's wrong, as his or her weight shows no improvement. Skipping meals never necessarily means that someone will gain weight. It just means that people who skip meals and gorge or overeat when it is mealtime won't see the desired effects.

MYTH: During fast periods, you literally can't eat anything.

TRUTH: This myth is partially true and partially false. It's true only for methods like 12:12, 14:10, 16:8, and 20:4 that require fasting and eating in alternation within each individual day. For 12:12 method, for example, you'd spend 12 hours fasting and 12 hours eating. In this case, you would definitely not eat anything or consume any calories during that 12-hour fasting window, but the same isn't true for methods that alternate between days "on" and days "off" between fasting and eating. For those types of methods, you absolutely can eat during fasting periods! It might feel counterintuitive as you read these words, but you don't explicitly have to eat nothing during fast periods. Most methods that have full days of fasting actually allow for caloric intake as long as it's restricted by 20-25% of one's normal intake. Therefore, for methods like 5:2, alternate-day, eat-stop-eat, and crescendo, on days when you're fasting, you can still consume around 500 calories, and that will help a lot!

MYTH: There's only one way to do IF that's right and truly the best.

TRUTH: This myth is absolutely and utterly false. There is no one right way to practice Intermittent Fasting, and part of the beauty of IF is that there are so many different methods, meaning each approaching IF likely has a few different options to choose from. Similarly, different body and personality types will be drawn to different methods, based on individuals' abilities and goals. IF is about flexibility, adjustment, and self-correction. There's no one right method for everyone, and there's no "best" method to strive for. Do whatever method feels right and suits your life, and once you've found it, practice it as long as you can! That's far more realistic and accessible.

MYTH: It's not natural to fast like that.

TRUTH: It's more natural to practice Intermittent Fasting than it is to eat three full meals each day! It's more connected to our evolutionary drives and to our primitive selves to eat like this. And it's better for our brains, hearts, cells, and digestive systems to have a break from food once in a while to recalibrate. As you learned in the Introduction, people have been practicing Intermittent Fasting as long as humans have been in existence. It's only myths like this that circulate today that make it seem like IF is foreign, unhealthy, and dangerous. Animals of all types become healthier after periods of fasting, and humans are no different. Remember that we are animals and that IF is in our nature. Proceed with that confidence and knowledge!

Chapter 11 Frequently Asked Questions

Most types of changes come with a lot of questions and intermittent fasting is no different. Here are some frequently asked questions from beginners.

Can I have coffee?

Yes, you can have black coffee, water, and plain steeped tea.

Can I add cream/sugar/milk in my coffee?

The goal of fasting is not to add calories, so the answer is no, you should not add anything to your coffee. However, I have heard of cases in which intermittent fasters add less than 50 calories to their coffee and they have claimed to still be successful with intermittent fasting; I have heard that it does not affect their fasted state, but keep in mind all individuals are not created equal. I would not recommend adding anything to your coffee, but if adding something to your coffee still makes this a good change for the goal you have for yourself, then give it a try.

Does intermittent fasting work well with veganism, paleo, keto, vegetarianism, or any other styles of eating?

Yes, the beauty of intermittent fasting is that it can be combined with any style of eating unless otherwise directed by a medical professional. You can turn your style of eating into the 16:8 method with ease, as this change does not restrict or state the style/types of food you eat, it is specifically based on the timing of your eating.

Is there an alternative to the 16:8 method if I cannot initially fast 16 hours and raise it up to 16?

Yes, especially for women, it is recommended that if women cannot or are not willing to do a 16 hour fast, they can start with a 14-hour fasting window and 10-hour feeding window. This is recommended for women, but men can start here if needed. Once the 14 hours is mastered, you can then work your way up to the 16:8 method.

Can I have a cheat meal?

Technically, you can eat what you want when intermittent fasting; there are no food group restrictions. There is no cheat meal to have, unless you have decided that you have put yourself on some type of restrictive meals/foods to not indulge in, if so, then yes, but I recommend to always eat in moderation.

What are some healthy snack foods to eat on the go during my feeding window?

Pepperoni slices, fruit, veggie tray, Skinny Pop popcorn individual bags (unless you will always measure the servings before consuming), turkey/beef jerky, individual peanut butter cups, whole grain cereal, almond milk, eggs, rice cakes, nuts (individual bags), hummus, and more.

I am too hungry during my fasting window. What should I do?

Be patient and your body to adapt to this change. This may take some time, for some, it occurs fast, for others, it may take a week or so, but this depends on how you were eating before you began this lifestyle. According to Collier in 2013, your body is still adjusting to how it was functioning before and is fighting you to get back to that way, as most people were eating more frequently and maybe even more meals or snacks during the day. Eventually, you will not feel this way. Eventually, you will adapt to your feeding and fasting windows and the urge to eat or the thought of starving will get easier and easier until it goes away.

Why am I not losing fat faster, like other people are?

It is more than likely a combination of not eating the appropriate portions when you are eating and/or not preparing to eat the right food choices. Although fat and weight loss can still happen, it is more frequent and visible when the appropriate food choices and portions are selected and prepared.

How can I stay full longer?

Eat more fiber and drink more water, stay hydrated.

Do I have to eat low carb?

No, you can eat what you want during your feeding window. I recommend eating proportionately and choosing healthier food options. Instead of white bread choose whole grain bread. Instead of white rice choose brown rice. Instead of anything with high fructose corn syrup, scratch it off, instead of canned fruit, eat fresh fruit.

Should I exercise in the fasted state?

You can, but it is not required. It is also not recommended on heavy lifting days.

What if I am on medications and must eat with my morning medications?

In this case, you would need to make your feeding window begin at whatever time you take your meds. I would recommend taking your meds as late as you can in the mornings but do get authorization of your plan from a medical professional.

Should I discuss this with my medical professional before beginning the change?

Yes, you should always discuss diet changes with a medical professional before you begin.

Frequent mistakes

People have failed due to the following frequent mistakes. Don't be one of these people, be knowledgeable and plan and think ahead.

One of the biggest mistakes beginners make is not finishing this book to the end and not taking this information seriously; basically, starting too soon, before you are prepared to start. While reading this book, it's a good idea to take notes, and jot down an individual plan while reading and sometimes doing further research during your reading. It wouldn't hurt even to read this book twice, especially if this is your first exposure to fasting, specifically intermittent fasting.

Another mistake that is made, not only with intermittent fasting but with any and most diet plans or lifestyle eating changes, is when people try to implement too many changes at once. Becoming a vegan and implementing intermittent fasting at the same time is not a great idea. Starting to work out with a trainer 4 days a week and implement intermittent fasting is not recommended. It is not goodstarting a new job with varying schedules and implement intermittent fasting at the same time. It is also nota good idea starting a new medication, a new workout plan, and intermittent fasting at the same time. Not to say this is impossible, it is, but on average these are too many changes at once for a beginner.

Most of us have been taught to eat 3 good sized meals a day, breakfast, lunch, and dinner (which includes dessert) and to have snacks in between meals, so anything outside of this set up seems out of the norm. Many people are habituated to always eating something during most times of their day. Most events we host or attend, are surrounded by food and beverages, so food is always readily available. Being without food for 16 hours sounds foreign and impossible because it is not what we are accustomed too.

Intermittent fasting brings about a new idea that life is not all about eating food all the time. People are in fear of this idea at the start, which denotes negativity; they may fail in making this big of a change due to their own negative assumptions and thoughts. Do not be afraid to be hungry; you will not starve during these 16 hours, you will survive, and be successful with weight loss, better health, and weight management.

During the beginning stages of intermittent fasting, it is vital to NOT constantly watch the clock. It is recommended that you use your time wisely. Intermittent fasting will inadvertently assist you with your time management if you listen to this recommendation. While fasting, be productive, stay busy, because 16 hours of fasting is just that 16 hours of not eating. Most people will sleep the majority of the 16 hours of fasting times, but it will take time for your body AND your mind to become accustomed to not eating breakfast or not eating or drinking whatever as soon as you wake up each morning, so make sure you attempt to stay busy and never get too much in your heard or get bored.

Some people are familiar with eating mostly junk foods: no nutrients, minerals, vitamins, or any form of a balanced meal. Sugar cravings, addictions, and food obsessiveness for these people will be one of your hardest challenges. A good way to counterbalance this is not to purchase sugary, unhealthy foods to be stored near you, especially during the beginning stages of intermittent fasting. We are accustomed to snacking all the time, snacking is allowed during the feeding windows, but it is recommended to make better snack options, choose fruit, not donuts, choose whole grain cereal instead of Frosted Flakes, choose nuts over candy bars.

Your body needs to be always hydrated. Sometimes your body sends your brain signals that it's hungry when you are not physically hungry; you are instead thirsty and needing liquid intake. A major mistake is not drinking an adequate amount of water daily. To assist with making water intake routine, people can start each meal with an 8 oz glass of water, drink steeped tea during either fasting or feeding times (both are acceptable), start the morning with a glass of lemon water, and/or during the feeding windows infuse water with fruits, mints, and more.

Lastly, but in no way least of the mistakes made by beginners is the idea that you don't need to choose your foods wisely. Yes, you can eat your favorite foods, yes you can still eat out at restaurants with your families, yes you can still attend social events which includes a buffet and more, but it is recommended to choose healthier options, use portion control, and read food labels if possible; basically, make smart choices to ensure you have optimal results while intermittent fasting. There is no diet or way of eating in which you can lose weight or maintain weight with no regard to calorie intake. Calories count no matter what diet or way of eating you are following. Intermittent fasting is no different; you cannot get away with excessive calorie intake.

Chapter 12 Hacks to Success

There are many principal tips and tricks that I use till this day to continue to ensure my success. While intermittent fasting is all about the timing of your meals and fasting, it can be so much more if you decide to use all the resources available to you to keep it exciting, continue to learn new things, be creative, be consistent and prepare and be always prepared. Intermittent fasting along with the hacks discussed below will change your weight and your life forever.

Sharing is Caring

I am not certain if this will help anyone other than myself or not, but it did help and is still helping me. I have learned that I am best at all things in life when I am helping others along the way. I have always shared my knowledge with people day in and day and have become a coach of intermittent fasting to many. By encouraging others, I have simultaneously helped myself, because it's a shame to teach what you can't follow right? I won't be that type of coach. I practice what I am teaching. Me writing this book has helped me learn that I know so much about this topic, which is why I have been so much more successful this time around.

Apps to Download

Pinterest is such a good resource to use when it comes to planning meals to keep eating the healthier way. This app includes links to recipes, grocery lists, meal idea, how to prep these meals, and more. YouTube, of course, is a great resource to review other people's struggles, peaks, and pits, before and after pictures, to hear their stories, to help you stay motivated and understand that most of what you go through while attempting to make this a habit, others have gone through the same things. MyFitnessPal's blog and community sections of its app is another great resource to use to join communities that are specific to intermittent fasting and all its components

These are good apps to have downloaded on your mobile device, iPad, or tablet. Using all your free time on these apps should be your new hobby instead of scrolling on your social media, especially since everything you see and hear will contribute to the success of making intermittent fasting a hobby.

Food Delivery Services

Some people decide that Meal Planning and Meal Prep is just not a realistic lifestyle for them. They may live a busier life than average, have a big active family, hate to cook, can't cook, don't want to cook, hate shopping, not creative, and more reasons. These people may choose to use a meal planning/prep or food delivery service to assist them with their meals.

Sometimes this can be costly, sometimes it may be affordable, but what it is, is convenient and by using this service you are still preparing in advance for what life throws at you during this change. You are still choosing healthier options, and being creative in what you eat.

Journaling

This lifestyle change will change your life forever. One day you will have changed so much that you may want to share your journey with others. If you decide to share, what better way to share than to go back and see how you felt each day or a few days. It is best practice to journal while you go through this journey. Journaling can be helpful in discovering what your negative triggers are, tracking your weight and measurement progress, tracking your feelings towards food, tracking your growth toward meal planning and food shopping and eating out and chosen food options, tracking your every step along the way. Your first journal entry should note why you are doing IF and explain your goals.

Sometimes people go as far as to go back to school for nutrition, or to be a trainer, life coach, and more, this journal will only assist you in tracking it all in real time. Your journal could be the road to success for someone or some other people who feel as though you once felt. This can also help you when you have those hard days and want to give up. Journaling can only help you on this journey; it is best practice for success.

Family Lifestyle Change

I wouldn't recommend making a drastic change, but after a few days maybe a week it's a good idea to start your family and sometimes even the company you keep around you to start eating what you eat and when you eat. If you are the cook and shopper in your house, this will be a better use of your time. You will only have to meal plan once, shop once, and cook a few meals that will feed everyone for a couple of days. Hopefully, this gives you more time during the week to add in exercise if you don't, or if you do maybe a second workout, or maybe give you a few hours of time each day to do something else you have been wanting to do, like maybe writing a book.

Brush your Teeth Earlier

Everyone should brush their teeth before bed each night. With intermittent fasting, it's better to practice brushing your teeth after your last meal. The taste of toothpaste and/orListerine should keep you from wanting to do any further eating. This is just a mind trick, but it has been a successful, helpful trick that I still use.

How to Order at Restaurants

Know the menu before you go. I repeat, know the menu before you go. Most restaurants, even fast-food restaurants, have websites in which you can view their menu options. If you know what's on the menu before you go, you can be proactive in deciding what you will order as the best option for you. Have a few staple times that most restaurants offer: grilled salmon, chicken breast, shrimp, any seafood, fried chicken wings no breading or sauce, burgers wrapped in lettuce, salads, and more.

Most restaurants DO NOT serve appropriate portions of food. This is an advertising mechanism for the restaurants; it is an effective way for them to get you to continually come back and spend money with them. I mean, who wants to go to a restaurant that serves those small plate options? Most restaurants serve 2 and sometimes 3 times the portion that a person should be eating in one sitting.

To ensure you spend your money wisely but getting the food you pay for, while simultaneously ensuring that you are using good portion control, when you order at a restaurant it is good practice to go ahead and ask for a to-go plate and when your food arrives, split your food up by keeping an appropriate portion to eat now and package away the other 2 or 3 servings for later options.

Lunch Bag Prep

Every evening after dinner, clean the kitchen and prepare for the next day. This includes preparing my lunch bag for the next day. I add the following to my lunch bag each day. 2 full meals, 3-4 snacks, and 2-3 bottles of water and sparkling water. Although most days, I eat dinner at home, what if I didn't make it home in time to eat dinner, or what if football practice goes long, what if traffic is a mess due to an accident, what if I must work late, what if, what if, what if. Always be prepared and you will be successful. I have had unplanned events, which have forced me to eat in the car, and sometimes dinner is a few healthy snacks because I didn't have my meal with me. Be prepared.

How to Deal with Unplanned Events

Although unplanned life events occur, sometimes 3-4 times a week, as an intermittent faster, you still need to have a plan for the unplanned. Always have that lunch box/bag with you as previously mentioned. Know a few staple food options that are your go-to food options when you are on the go and don't have your own available food options. Think before you eat always.

Peer pressure is real, especially at social events, be sure to have a serious conversation with family and friends so they know you are serious and that they should not offer you items when it is not your feeding window and that your new lifestyle is not a joking matter and that you would appreciate they take it as an important part of your life. Make good decisions and be proud of those decisions that you make. Every now and then, I change my feeding windows for social events. I sometimes fast longer so that I can push my feeding window back to be able to attend social events and have dinner and drinks with family and friends.

Buy in Bulk

You may be thinking how is buying in buck related to intermittent fasting. It is vital for beginners and sometimes longtime intermittent fasters to always have food on hand to accommodate any cravings and their feeding windows. It is best practice to buy favorite snack foods in bulk if available. When you buy these items in bulk you can then use small Ziplock and/or sandwich bags to create your own individual serving size (according to the food label) baggies to keep in your car, purse, backpack, at school, at work, in your gym bag, in your lunch box or bag, and more.

It saves you money buying in bulk than to buy individual items already prepackage, companies charge more for convenience, so when you buy prepackaged small cute individually packaged items, it costs more than buying in bulk and doing this yourself. This also ensures that you are only having a serving or 2 according to the food label. This also saves you from not being prepared and eating unplanned food items.

Consistent Routine

Appetite is trainable because it is driven by routine. Our bodies know and learn our routines, we are usually hungry when we expect to be hungry, not necessarily when we are physically hunger, again it could be that we are bored or need fluids. Practice makes perfect, right? Fasting is a skill that with intermittent fasting, you are trying to advance this skill.

Best practice would be at least start with a good routine new life as you endure this lifestyle change. That means to set your alarm and wake to start most days at the same time, specifically during the week to start. Eat your first meal and the second meal at the same times; you can have your snacks at whatever time during the feeding window. It is also best practice to workout at the same time of the day most days and take measurements, pictures, and weigh yourself on these same days. Meal plan the week before you will shop and cook the meals. Then shop on the same day, and cook and prep the meals on the same day so you start the week always with good habits.

Setbacks

Setbacks are sometimes inevitable when it comes to any type of life change; intermittent fasting is no different. Setbacks can include general fasting knowledge, lack of discipline, willpower, self-control, fear of missing out, lack of planning or procrastination, illnesses, that may or may not include medications, that prevent this type of fasting, lack of motivation, resistance to change, YOU, and much more.

YOU

You will be your biggest setback, challenge, and critic during this attempt to change. Many people have issues with confidence, self-esteem, feeling deserving, discipline, consistency, peer pressure, unawareness, and more, which ALL can contribute to YOU being your worst nightmare during this change and ultimately maybe your demise in many aspects of life.

You must realize you are the only person who can make a change in your life, and that goes for all the changes you want to make. You are responsible for your own happiness and if changing your eating lifestyle is what will make you happier, then this information gives you the knowledge to be able to make this change without help from anyone else. You can make this change happen for YOU, and only you. You should be beginning this journal to please only you and not just for appearance purposes, but for through and through happiness and well-being.

You must believe in yourself. You must know that you are your #1 priority and must be your biggest supporter. If no one else cares, you must care enough to change your habits and be consistent in the changes you decide to make. No one should be able to derail you from making such an important change in your life.

You are responsible for your choices. This is a lifestyle change, so if you mess up, just do better the next time, don't quit on yourself. Don't make decisions based on temporary needs or feelings; think about what you do as you do it to make decisions that are better for you overall in the future. Think about your future, do you want to be trying another diet in another 30 days? Do you still want to be in the same body with the same health in 30 days? Would you rather feel comfortable in your clothes and skin and feel healthy throughout?

Practice Makes Perfect

Getting acquainted with the process of fasting in general and testing your chosen time frames for your feeding and fasting windows can be a difficult time if you are used to eating many meals/snacks daily. Being motivated to continue to develop in this change is just as important as anything else that comes along with this change. Live each day separately, as in if something did not go to your liking one day, change your process the next until you have feeding and fasting windows that work well with your daily routine schedule. Mind over matter, you matter, so make sure your mind continues to know this fact to ensure you aren't resistant to this change.

Don't be Weak

During the initial change stage, there must be an increased amount of willpower, discipline, and self-control. You will be required to practice your self-control around others who are NOT on an intermittent fasting lifestyle. You need to have the willpower to refrain from ingesting calories during their fasting window. You need to have the discipline to create these time frames and stick to them, and when the feeding and/or fasting windows are broken, create consequences for yourself to ensure it does not happen again until it does not happen anymore.

Fear of Missing Out (FOMO)

Because of how you are used to living your life, sometimes you may feel like you are missing out on the fun surrounding social and/or family eating events, but consider the fact that you are making this change to perfect how you feel and how you look to ensure you are around for a long life to enjoy life. Family and friends may not be on this lifestyle and either will or will not support this change. Alcohol should be consumed in moderation. If you choose to drink alcohol, two or less daily drinks should be the max. Choose non-sugary spirits and alcohol volume dry wines to ensure you are getting the best buzz for your choice.

Holidays will more than likely be the biggest change for you and the biggest day to test you when new to this lifestyle. Holidays are all about eating and tasting everything with family and friends and making memories. Try to prepare in advance by either assisting with cooking to ensure meals are ready before/during your feeding window and choose your favorites to ensure you are satisfied and not as vulnerable after your feeding window closes. The holidays will test you.

Prepare, Don't Procrastinate

Preparation is key. Now that you have decided on your feeding window, ALWAYS, make sure you have your meals/snacks readily available during these times. Stay ahead of your schedule a day or so, to ensure you pack your meals/snacks if you are away from home when it is time to eat those meals/snacks to ensure. Even if you plan to be home, always make sure you take at least a few snack options with your wherever you go, by preparing in this way you ensure not to ever get caught out and about for hours with nothing to eat just wasting your feeding window away.

Not Reading Labels and Controlling Portions

Although your calories are NOT restricted when intermittent fasting, eating too much of even healthy foods can lead to weight gain no matter the type of diet/lifestyle you are following. To prevent this type of setback meal plan, use portion control, be consistent with choosing the most nutritious food choices, and measure your foods to ensure you are not eating too many servings in one meal.

Nonsense from Others

There are times in life when it's better to keep your goals to yourself. Keep your goals away from negative people, specifically keep negative people away from your goals and out of your life. To be successful in many things in life, you need a support system, which does not include negative people. You need someone who can cheer you on, someone who can motivate you, someone, who may be willing to join you, someone who doesn't add to your problems by persuading you to do what is against your goals. If you have these types of people in your life, do not tell them your plan of intermittent fasting.

Many people have their own preconceived assumptions about fasting, and intermittent fasting, and usually their views are without researched knowledge and education. It is important that you understand and know myth versus facts when it comes to intermittent fasting. People who have tried all types of diets seem to think they know them all, and they are very discouraging at times. During a lifestyle change as intermittent fasting, it is very easy to get discouraged, so stay the course and keep those people away, while you try this out yourself based on your researched facts.

Chapter 13 Recipes

BREAKFAST

Breakfast Cherry Muffins

Preparation Time: 10 minutes

Cooking Time: 30 minutes

Servings: 6

Ingredients:

1 ½ cup almond flour

¼ cup arrowroot flour

¼ cup coconut oil

¼ cup maple syrup

3 whole eggs

2 teaspoons vanilla extract

1 ½ teaspoons almond extract

1 teaspoon baking powder

1 cup fresh cherry, pitted and chopped

¼ teaspoon salt

Directions:

Preheat the oven to 350ᵒF.

In a mixing bowl, combine all ingredients except for the cherries. Mix until well-combined.

Add the cherries last.

Fill muffin liners with the batter and bake for 30 minutes or until a toothpick inserted comes out clean.

Nutrition:

Calories 528, Total Fat 39g, Saturated Fat 5g, Total Carbs 36g, Net Carbs 29g, Protein 13g, Sugar: 15g, Fiber: 7g, Sodium: 177mg, Potassium 679mg

Breakfast Shakshuka

Preparation Time: 5 minutes

Cooking Time: 10 minutes

Servings: 6

Ingredients:

1 tablespoon olive oil

½ onion, chopped

1 clove garlic, minced

1 red bell pepper, seeded and chopped

4 cups tomatoes, diced

1 teaspoon chili powder

1 teaspoon paprika

6 eggs, pasture-raised

½ tablespoon fresh parsley, chopped

salt and pepper to taste

Directions:

Heat oil in a skillet over medium flame.

Sauté the onion and garlic for 30 seconds or until fragrant.

Add in the red bell pepper and tomatoes. Season with salt and pepper to taste. Stir in the chili powder and paprika. Allow to simmer until the tomatoes are soft.

Reduce the heat and create 6 wells in the skillet.

Crack in one egg in each well and increase the heat.

Cover and allow to simmer for 5 minutes.

Garnish with parsley last.

Nutrition:

Calories 177, Total Fat 12g, Saturated Fat 3g, Total Carbs 7g, Net Carbs 5g, Protein 10g, Sugar: 4g, Fiber: 2g, Sodium:109 mg, Potassium 445mg

Keto Crepes

Preparation Time: 5 minutes

Cooking Time: 4 minutes

Servings: 4

Ingredients:

2 tablespoon coconut flour

4 large eggs, pasture-raised

1 tablespoon coconut oil

1 cup hazelnuts, soaked in water overnight

2/3 cup dark chocolates

½ teaspoon vanilla extract

2 tablespoon maple syrup

½ cup water

Directions:

Preheat the oven to 3500F.

In a bowl, mix the coconut flour, eggs, and water until well-combined.

Heat oil in a skillet over medium flame and grease the skillet with coconut oil.

Scoop 1/3 cup of the crepe mixture into the skillet and cook for 4 minutes while flipping halfway through the cooking time.

Repeat until all batter is made into crepes.

Make the hazelnut sauce by combining the hazelnuts, dark chocolates, vanilla extract, and maple syrup in a blender.

Pulse until smooth.

Spread the Nutella sauce over the crepes before serving.

Nutrition:

Calories 465, Total Fat 29g, Saturated Fat 6g, Total Carbs 46g, Net Carbs g, Protein 9g, Sugar: 32g, Fiber: 5g, Sodium: 53mg, Potassium 401mg

Blueberry Hemp Seed Smoothie

Preparation Time: 5 minutes

Cooking Time: 0 minutes

Servings: 1

Ingredients:

1 ¼ cup frozen blueberries

2 tablespoons hemp seeds

1 serving vanilla plant-based protein powder

½ cup packed fresh spinach

1 teaspoon spirulina powder

1 ¼ unsweetened plant-based milk

¼ teaspoon holy basil leaves, chopped

Directions:

Place all ingredients in a blender.

Blend until smooth.

Nutrition:

Calories 442, Total Fat 19g, Saturated Fat 5g, Total Carbs 50g, Net Carbs 43g, Protein 27g, Sugar: 33g, Fiber: 7g, Sodium: 426mg, Potassium 960mg

Chickpea Scramble with Kale

Preparation Time: 5 minutes

Cooking Time: 5 minutes

Servings: 2

Ingredients:
1 cup chickpea flour

1 teaspoon turmeric powder

1 tablespoon nutritional yeast

1 tablespoon olive oil

½ small onion, diced

4 cloves of garlic, minced

1 bunch kale, torn into small pieces

½ cup water

½ teaspoon salt

Directions:

Mix the chickpea flour and water until well-combined. Season with salt, turmeric powder, and nutritional yeast.

Heat oil in a skillet over medium flame.

Sauté the onion and garlic until fragrant.

Stir in the kale for 30 seconds.

Pour in the chickpea mixture and continue mixing for 3 minutes or until the chickpea eggs have set.

Nutrition:

Calories 279, Total Fat10 g, Saturated Fat 1g, Total Carbs 34g, Net Carbs 27g, Protein 14g, Sugar: 6g, Fiber: 7g, Sodium: 301mg, Potassium 698mg

Quick and Creamy Whole Grain Porridge

Preparation Time: 5 minutes

Cooking Time: 5 minutes

Servings: 2

Ingredients:

½ cup cooked quinoa

¼ cup sunflower seeds

¼ cup raw walnuts

2 tablespoons chopped dates

1 teaspoon cinnamon

¼ cup almond milk

1 tablespoon raw honey

½ diced apple

1 tablespoon chia seeds

Directions:

In a saucepan, add the quinoa, sunflower seeds, walnuts, dates, cinnamon, milk, and raw honey.

Heat over medium flame. Add more water or water to achieve a porridge consistency.

Before serving, stir in apple and chia seeds last.

Nutrition:

Calories 317, Total Fat 17g, Saturated Fat 2g, Total Carbs 39g, Net Carbs 33g, Protein 8g, Sugar: 22g, Fiber: 6g, Sodium: 27mg, Potassium 365mg

Omega-3 Chocolate Chia Hemp Pudding

Preparation Time: 5 minutes

Cooking Time: 0 minutes

Servings: 1

Ingredients:

2 tablespoons chia seeds

2 tablespoons hemp seeds

1 tablespoon cacao powder

6 small pitted dates, chopped

½ cup unsweetened almond milk

½ teaspoon pure vanilla extract

1 tablespoon chocolate protein powder

¼ teaspoon salt

Directions:

Add all ingredients in a blender and pulse until smooth.

Pour into individual containers and place inside the fridge for at least 2 hours before serving.

Nutrition:

Calories 367, Total Fat 13g, Saturated Fat 1g, Total Carbs 55 g, Net Carbs 47g, Protein 12g, Sugar: 39g, Fiber: 8g, Sodium: 129mg, Potassium 686mg

No Bake Granola Breakfast Bars

Preparation Time: 2 hours 15 minutes

Cooking Time: 0 minutes

Servings: 6

Ingredients:

2 cups raisins, soaked in water then drained

3 tablespoons pure maple syrup

½ cup tahini or almond butter

2 cups oats

1 cup raw sunflower seeds

½ cup cacao nibs

Directions:

Mix all ingredients in mixing bowl until well-combined.

Press firmly into a parchment-lined baking pan.

Allow to set in the fridge for two hours.

Remove from the pan once set and slice into bars.

Nutrition:

Calories 372, Total Fat 26g, Saturated Fat 3g, Total Carbs 36g, Net Carbs 27g, Protein 15g, Sugar: 9g, Fiber: 9g, Sodium: 52mg, Potassium 511mg

Keto Energy Bars

Preparation Time: 15 minutes

Cooking Time: 0 minutes

Servings: 5

Ingredients:

1 ¼ cup packed dates, pitted and chopped

1 cup unsweetened fine coconut meat

1 cup hemp seeds

2/3 cup cashew nuts, toasted and chopped

2 tablespoons coconut oil

Directions:

 Place all ingredients in a food processor until well-combined.

Line a baking dish with parchment paper and press the dough into the pan.

Place in the fridge for an hour to set.

Once frozen, lift the bars out of the pan and cut into 10 squares.

Nutrition:

Calories 471, Total Fat 34g, Saturated Fat 6g, Total Carbs 41g, Net Carbs 34g, Protein 10g, Sugar: 26g, Fiber: 7g, Sodium:60 mg, Potassium 588mg

No-Bake Chocolate Chia Energy Bars

Preparation Time: 10 minutes

Cooking Time: 0 minutes

Servings: 5

Ingredients:

1 ½ cups pitted dates, chopped

1/3 cup cacao powder

½ cup whole chia seeds

½ cup shredded coconut

1 cup raw walnut, chopped

½ cup dark chocolate bar, chopped

½ cup oats

½ teaspoon vanilla extract

¼ teaspoon salt

Directions:

Place all ingredients in a food processor and pulse until a thick dough is formed.

Line a baking pan with parchment paper.

Press the dough into the pan.

Place inside the fridge to allow to set for at least 2 hours.

Once hardened, slice into 10 bars.

Nutrition:

Calories 284, Total Fat 12g, Saturated Fat 1g, Total Carbs 45g, Net Carbs g, Protein 5g, Sugar: 32g, Fiber: 6g, Sodium: 40mg, Potassium 506mg

Breakfast Oatmeal Raisin Bars

Preparation Time: 2 hours 15 minutes

Cooking Time: 0 minutes

Servings: 8

Ingredients:

3 cups dates, pitted and chopped

2 cups oats

½ cup chocolate chips, organic

½ cup raisins

½ teaspoon salt

Directions:

Place all ingredients in a food processor and pulse until a thick dough is formed.

Line a baking pan with parchment paper.

Press the dough into the pan.

Place inside the fridge to allow to set for at least 2 hours.

Once hardened, slice into 16 bars.

Nutrition:

Calories 235, Total Fat 3g, Saturated Fat 1g, Total Carbs 59g, Net Carbs 51g, Protein 6g, Sugar: 36g, Fiber: 8g, Sodium: 3mg, Potassium 520 mg

Tropical Chia Seed Oats

Preparation Time: 2 hours 15 minutes

Cooking Time: 0 minutes

Servings: 1

Ingredients:

½ cup quick oats

1 cup diced fresh pineapples

1 tablespoon chia seeds

1 cup unsweetened almond milk

½ teaspoon pure vanilla extract

1 sliced banana

2 tablespoons toasted coconut

Directions:

In a container, place the oats, pineapples, chia seeds, almond milk, and vanilla. Stir to combine everything.

Place inside the fridge for at least 2 hours.

Once ready, top with banana and toasted coconut.

Nutrition:

Calories 535, Total Fat 14g, Saturated Fat 4g, Total Carbs 89g, Net Carbs76 g, Protein 17g, Sugar: 42g, Fiber: 13g, Sodium: 142mg, Potassium 1129mg

Quinoa Breakfast Bowl

Preparation Time: 10 minutes

Cooking Time: 15 minutes

Servings: 1

Ingredients:

¼ cup quinoa, rinsed

2 tablespoons dried goji berries

1 small banana, peeled and sliced

¼ cup fresh blueberries

1 tablespoon chopped walnuts

1 tablespoon slivered almonds

1 tablespoon pumpkin seeds, hulled

¼ cup unsweetened almond milk

1 tablespoon maple syrup

1/8 teaspoon ground cinnamon

1/8 teaspoon vanilla extract

¾ cup water

Directions:

Bring water to a boil in a small pot and add quinoa. Cook for 12 to 15 minutes then drain.

Allow the quinoa to cool. Fluff it and place in a bowl.

Top with goji berries, banana, blueberries, walnuts, almond, and pumpkin seed.

Pour over almond milk and maple syrup.

Dust with cinnamon and flavor with vanilla extract.

Nutrition:
Calories 516, Total Fat 13g, Saturated Fat 1g, Total Carbs 94g, Net Carbs 85g, Protein 13g, Sugar: 47g, Fiber: 9g, Sodium: 70mg, Potassium 949mg

Quinoa Bowls Avocado Egg

Preparation Time: 10 minutes

Cooking Time: 10 minutes

Servings: 1

Ingredients:
2 teaspoons extra virgin olive oil

2 large eggs, pasture-raised

1 cup grape tomatoes, halve

1 teaspoon red wine vinegar

1 cup cooked quinoa

½ cup black beans, cooked

2 tablespoons chopped cilantro

½ ripe avocado, sliced

What you'll need from the store cupboard:
¼ teaspoon salt

Directions:
Heat oil in a skillet over medium flame.

Fry the eggs for 3 minutes. Set aside.

Using the same skillet, sauté the tomatoes for 3 minutes until wilted.

Add in the red wine vinegar and season with salt and pepper to taste. Set aside.

Assemble the bowl by putting the quinoa in a bowl and top with beans and tomatoes. Add in the eggs and avocado.

Garnish with avocado slices.

Nutrition:

Calories 343, Total Fat 16g, Saturated Fat 3.1 g, Total Carbs 35g, Net Carbs 26g, Protein 15g, Sugar: 3g, Fiber: 9g, Sodium: 332mg, Potassium 893mg

Keto Porridge

Preparation Time: 2 hours and 10 minutes

Cooking Time: 10 minutes

Servings: 2

Ingredients:

2 tablespoons hemp seeds

¼ cup walnuts, chopped

¼ cup toasted coconuts

¼ cup unsweetened almond milk

¼ cup coconut milk

¼ cup almond butter

1 tablespoon extra-virgin coconut oil

¼ teaspoon ground turmeric

1 teaspoon bee pollen

¼ teaspoon cinnamon

2 tablespoons chia seeds

Directions:

Roast the hemp seeds, walnuts, and coconuts in a skillet until toasted. Set aside.

In the same skillet, heat the almond milk, coconut milk, and almond butter until everything is combined. Set aside and allow to cool.

To the milk mixture, add in the coconut oil, turmeric, bee pollen, and cinnamon.

Assemble the porridge by putting the toasted nuts at the bottom of the bowl.

Add in chia seeds.

: Pour in the milk mixture.

Allow to soak in the fridge for at least 2 hours.

Nutrition:

Calories 575, Total Fat 50g, Saturated Fat 4g, Total Carbs 6g, Net Carbs 4g, Protein 15g, Sugar: 4g, Fiber: 2g, Sodium: 57mg, Potassium 645 mg

Ginger Turmeric Oatmeal

Preparation Time: 8 hours and 5 minutes

Cooking Time: 0 minutes

Servings: 2

Ingredients:

1 cup rolled oats

2 tablespoons maple syrup

¼ teaspoon ground turmeric

¼ teaspoon ground ginger

1 cup frozen assorted berries

½ cup water

A pinch of black of pepper

Directions:

Mix the oats with water, maple, turmeric, black pepper, and ginger until well-combined.

Add in the berries.

Allow to sit in the fridge overnight.

Nutrition:

Calories 280, Total Fat 6g, Saturated Fat 3g, Total Carbs 64g, Net Carbs 57g, Protein 11g, Sugar: 30g, Fiber: 7g, Sodium: 59mg, Potassium 456mg

LUNCH

Spinach Soup

Preparation time: *10 minutes*

Cooking time: *20 minutes*

Servings: *4*

Ingredients:

4 cups vegetable stock

1 pound spinach leaves

½ teaspoon sweet paprika

1 teaspoon cumin, ground

2 tablespoons avocado oil

4 scallions, chopped

2 tomatoes, cubed

A pinch of salt and black pepper

2 teaspoons lime juice

1 tablespoon parsley, chopped

Directions:

Heat up a pot with the oil over medium heat, add the scallions and the tomatoes and sauté for 5 minutes.
Add the spinach, paprika and the other ingredients, bring to a simmer and cook over medium heat for 15 minutes more.
Divide the soup into bowls and serve.

Nutrition: calories 98, fat 4.1, fiber 1.7, carbs 13.1, protein 4.1

Mushroom Stew

Preparation time: *5 minutes*

Cooking time: *25 minutes*

Servings: *4*

Ingredients:

1 pound mushrooms, halved

2 scallions, chopped

2 garlic cloves, minced

2 tablespoons olive oil

2 tomatoes, cubed

1 cup vegetable stock

1 teaspoon turmeric powder

½ teaspoon cayenne pepper

A pinch of salt and black pepper

½ teaspoon hot paprika

½ teaspoon red pepper flakes, crushed

1 tablespoon dill, chopped

Directions:

Heat up a pot with the oil over medium heat, add the scallions and the garlic and sauté for 2 minutes.

Add the turmeric, cayenne and hot paprika and cook for 2 minutes more.

Add the mushrooms and sauté them for 1 more minute.

Add the rest of the ingredients, toss cook over medium heat for 20 minutes, divide into bowls and serve.

Nutrition: calories 108, fat 8.1, fiber 2.5, carbs 8.8, protein 4.6

Asparagus Soup

Preparation time: *10 minutes*

Cooking time: *20 minutes*

Servings: *4*

Ingredients:

2 garlic cloves, minced

2 tablespoons avocado oil

1 bunch asparagus, trimmed and halved

1 cup coconut cream

2 scallions, chopped

3 cups vegetable stock

½ teaspoon nutmeg, ground

½ teaspoons rosemary, dried

A pinch of salt and black pepper

Directions:

Heat up a pot with the oil over medium heat, add the scallions and the garlic and sauté for 5 minutes.
Add the asparagus and the other ingredients except the cream, stir, bring to a simmer and cook over medium heat for 15 minutes.
Add the cream, blend the soup using an immersion blender, divide into bowls and serve.

Nutrition: calories 161, fat 15.9, fiber 2.5, carbs 6.5, protein 2.3

Green Beans and Leeks Soup

Preparation time: *10 minutes*

Cooking time: *25 minutes*

Servings: *4*

Ingredients:

4 leeks, sliced

6 cups vegetable stock

1 tablespoon avocado oil

1 pound green beans, trimmed and halved

1 tablespoon cilantro, chopped

A pinch of salt and black pepper

1 teaspoon turmeric powder

½ teaspoon chili powder

1 tablespoon chives, chopped

Directions:

Heat up a pot with the oil over medium heat, add the leeks, turmeric and chili powder and sauté for 5 minutes. Add the green beans and the other ingredients except the chives, toss, bring to a simmer and cook over medium heat for 20 minutes stirring from time to time. Ladle the soup into bowls, sprinkle the chives on top and serve.

Nutrition: calories 97, fat 1, fiber 5.9, carbs 21.5, protein 3.6

Garlicky Endives Soup

Preparation time: *10 minutes*

Cooking time: *25 minutes*

Servings: *4*

Ingredients:

2 endives, shredded

2 scallions, chopped

3 garlic cloves, minced

2 tablespoons avocado oil

4 cups vegetable stock

A pinch of salt and black pepper

1 cup coconut cream

1 tablespoon coriander, chopped

½ teaspoon cumin, ground

½ teaspoon rosemary, dried

Directions:

Heat up a pot with the oil over medium heat, add the scallions, garlic, coriander, cumin and the rosemary, stir and sauté for 5 minutes.

Add the endives and the other ingredients, bring to a simmer, and cook over medium heat for 20 minutes more.

Blend using an immersion blender, divide into bowls and serve.

Nutrition: calories 140, fat 2, fiber 1, carbs 5, protein 10

Green Beans Stew

Preparation time: *10 minutes*

Cooking time: *25 minutes*

Servings: *4*

Ingredients:

1 pound green beans, trimmed and halved

2 cups vegetable stock

2 spring onions, chopped

1 tablespoon olive oil

2 garlic cloves, minced

½ teaspoon cumin, ground

½ teaspoon rosemary, dried

1 teaspoon garam masala

½ cup tomato passata

A pinch of salt and black pepper

1 tablespoon cilantro, chopped

Directions:

Heat up a pot with the oil over medium heat, add the spring onions, garlic, cumin, rosemary and garam masala, stir and sauté for 5 minutes

Add the green beans and the other ingredients, toss and cook everything for 20 minutes more.

Divide the stew into bowls and serve.

Nutrition: calories 93, fat 3.7, fiber 5.9, carbs 13.7, protein 4.1

Kale Soup

Preparation time: *10 minutes*

Cooking time: *25 minutes*

Servings: *4*

Ingredients:

2 tablespoons avocado oil

1 pound kale, torn

2 garlic cloves

1 teaspoon sweet paprika

1 teaspoon rosemary, dried

4 cups vegetable stock

1 cup coconut cream

1 tablespoon cilantro, chopped

A pinch of salt and black pepper

Directions:

Heat up a pot with the oil over medium heat, add the garlic, rosemary and the paprika and sauté for 5 minutes Add the kale, the stock and the other ingredients, bring to a simmer and cook over medium heat for 20 minutes. Divide into bowls and serve.

Nutrition: calories 192, fat 18.8, fiber 1.2, carbs 5.1, protein 3.2

Cabbage and Tomato Soup

Preparation time: *10 minutes*

Cooking time: *25 minutes*

Servings: *4*

Ingredients:

2 shallots, chopped

1 tablespoon avocado oil

½ pound cherry tomatoes, halved

1 green cabbage head, shredded

1 tablespoon basil, chopped

5 cups vegetable stock

½ teaspoon chili powder

½ teaspoon sweet paprika

1 teaspoon lime juice

A pinch of salt and black pepper

1 tablespoon cilantro, chopped

Directions:

Heat up a pot with the oil over medium high heat, add the shallots, chili powder and paprika and sauté for 5 minutes.
Add the cabbage, the stock and the other ingredients, toss and cook over medium heat for 20 minutes more.
Divide the soup into bowls and serve.

Nutrition: calories 89, fat 3.8, fiber 5.1, carbs 13.5, protein 2.9

Balsamic Bok Choy and Green Beans

Preparation time: *10 minutes*

Cooking time: *25 minutes*

Servings: *4*

Ingredients:

1 tablespoon avocado oil

1 pound bok choy, torn

½ pound green beans, trimmed and halved

2 garlic cloves, minced

2 scallions, chopped

½ teaspoon cayenne pepper

½ teaspoon turmeric powder

A pinch of salt and black pepper

½ cup vegetable stock

1 tablespoon balsamic vinegar

1 tablespoon cilantro, chopped

Directions:

Heat up a pan with the oil over medium heat, add the garlic, scallions, cayenne and turmeric and sauté for 5 minutes.

Add the bok choy, green beans and the other ingredients, bring to a simmer and cook over medium heat for 20 minutes more.

Divide everything between plates and serve for lunch.

Nutrition: calories 150, fat 12, fiber 2, carbs 4, protein 8

Fennel and Tomatoes Stew

Preparation time: *10 minutes*

Cooking time: *20 minutes*

Servings: 4

Ingredients:

1 pound cherry tomatoes, halved

2 fennel bulbs, sliced

1 cup tomato passata

1 cup vegetable stock

1 teaspoon red pepper flakes, crushed

2 shallots, chopped

1 tablespoon olive oil

1 tablespoon balsamic vinegar

A pinch of salt and black pepper

1 teaspoon rosemary, dried

1 teaspoon fennel powder

1 tablespoon cilantro, chopped

Directions:

Heat up a pot with the oil over medium heat, add the shallots, fennel, pepper flakes and fennel powder and sauté for 5 minutes.

Add the tomatoes and the other ingredients, bring to a simmer and cook over heat for 15 minutes.

Divide the stew into bowls and serve for lunch.

Nutrition: calories 120, fat 8, fiber 1, carbs 3, protein 7

Sesame Red Cabbage and Chives

Preparation time: *5 minutes*

Cooking time: *20 minutes*

Servings: *4*

Ingredients:

2 garlic cloves, minced

2 tablespoons avocado oil

1 tablespoon balsamic vinegar

2 spring onions, chopped

1 red cabbage head, shredded

½ cup tomato passata

1 tablespoon sesame seeds

1 tablespoon chives, chopped

Directions:

Heat up a pan with the oil over medium heat, add the garlic and spring onions and sauté for 5 minutes
Add the cabbage and the rest of the ingredients, toss, cook over medium heat for 15 minutes more, divide between plates and serve for lunch.

Nutrition: calories 120, fat 3, fiber 1, carbs 3, protein 6

Artichokes Chili

Preparation time: *10 minutes*

Cooking time: *20 minutes*

Servings: *4*

Ingredients:

1 tablespoon chili powder

10 ounces canned artichoke hearts, drained and halved

1 tablespoon avocado oil

2 scallions, chopped

½ cup vegetable stock

2 shallots, chopped

1 teaspoon hot paprika

½ teaspoon rosemary, dried

A pinch of salt and black pepper

1 tablespoon lime juice

1 tablespoon cilantro, chopped

Directions:

Heat up a pot with the oil over medium high heat, add the scallions, shallots, paprika and chili powder and sauté for 5 minutes.

Add the artichokes and the other ingredients, toss and cook over medium heat for 15 minutes more.

Divide the chili into bowls and serve.

Nutrition: calories 245, fat 12.2, fiber 1, carbs 5, protein 1.2

Green Beans Soup

Preparation time: *10 minutes*

Cooking time: *25 minutes*

Servings: 6

Ingredients:

1 tablespoon olive oil

2 spring onions, chopped

1 pound green beans, trimmed and halved

4 cups vegetable stock

1 teaspoon smoked paprika

A pinch of red pepper flakes

2 tomatoes, cubed

2 tablespoons lime juice

A pinch of salt and black pepper

Directions:

Heat up a pot with the oil over medium high heat, add the spring onions, pepper flakes and the paprika and sauté for 5 minutes

Add the green beans and the other ingredients, bring to a simmer and cook over medium heat for 20 minutes more.

Ladle the soup into bowls and serve.

Nutrition: calories 150, fat 3, fiber 2, carbs 4, protein 8

Broccoli Soup

Preparation time: *10 minutes*

Cooking time: *25 minutes*

Servings: *4*

Ingredients:

1 pound broccoli florets

2 spring onions, chopped

1 teaspoon chili powder

½ teaspoon coriander, ground

1 cup coconut cream

1 quart vegetable stock

A pinch of salt and black pepper

2 teaspoons ginger, grated

1 tablespoon cilantro, chopped

Directions:

Put the stock into a pot, bring to a simmer over medium heat, add the broccoli, spring onions and the other ingredients except the cream and cilantro, bring to a simmer and cook for 25 minutes.

Add the cream, blend the soup using an immersion blender, divide into bowls and serve with the cilantro sprinkled on top.

Nutrition: calories 140, fat 2, fiber 1, carbs 3, protein 7

Avocado Cream

Preparation time: *10 minutes*

Cooking time: *0 minutes*

Servings: *4*

Ingredients:

½ teaspoon coriander, ground

2 shallots, chopped

2 big avocados, peeled, pitted and chopped

1 tablespoon ginger, grated

4 cups vegetable stock

1 cup coconut cream

A pinch of salt and black pepper

1 tablespoon cilantro, chopped

Directions:

1. In a blender, combine the avocados with the coriander, stock and the other ingredients, pulse well, divide into bowls and serve.

Nutrition: calories 302, fat 29.5, fiber 6.5, carbs 12.1, protein 3.1

Oregano Olives Stew

Preparation time: *10 minutes*

Cooking time: *20 minutes*

Servings: *4*

Ingredients:

1 cup black olives, pitted and halved

1 cup kalamata olives, pitted and halved

1 tablespoon olive oil

2 shallots, chopped

1 cup tomato passata

1 cup coconut cream

A pinch of salt and black pepper

1 tablespoon oregano, chopped

Directions:

Heat up a pan with the oil over medium heat, add the shallots and the oregano sauté for 5 minutes.
Add the olives and the other ingredients, toss, bring to a simmer and cook over medium heat for 15 minutes more.
Divide into bowls and serve for lunch.

Nutrition: calories 130, fat 7.1, fiber 1, carbs 5.2, protein 3

Baked Paprika Cabbage Mix

Preparation time: *10 minutes*

Cooking time: *20 minutes*

Servings: *4*

Ingredients:

1 green cabbage head, roughly shredded

½ cup coconut cream

1 tablespoon avocado oil

1 tablespoon sweet paprika

1 tablespoon tomato passata

2 garlic cloves, minced

A pinch of salt and black pepper

1 tablespoon chives, chopped

Directions:

In a roasting pan, combine the cabbage with the oil, paprika and the other ingredients, toss, and bake at 370 degrees F for 20 minutes

Divide between plates and serve for lunch.

Nutrition: calories 120, fat 2, fiber 2, carbs 5, protein 8

Baked Turmeric Asparagus

Preparation time: *10 minutes*

Cooking time: *20 minutes*

Servings: *4*

Ingredients:

1 tablespoon avocado oil

2 bunches of asparagus, trimmed

1 teaspoon turmeric powder

½ cup vegetable stock

1 teaspoon chili powder

1 teaspoon coriander, ground

2 tablespoons lime juice

1 tablespoon cashew cheese, shredded

A pinch of salt and black pepper

Directions:

Arrange the asparagus on a baking sheet lined with parchment paper, add the oil, turmeric and the other ingredients, toss and bake at 390 degrees F for 20 minutes.
Divide the mix between plates and serve for lunch.

Nutrition: calories 160, fat 7, fiber 2, carbs 6, protein 10

Asparagus and Coconut Sauce

Preparation time: *10 minutes*

Cooking time: *20 minutes*

Servings: *4*

Ingredients:

¼ cup scallions, chopped

1 pound asparagus, trimmed and halved

1 cup coconut cream

1 teaspoon turmeric powder

2 garlic cloves, minced

1 tablespoon pine nuts, toasted

1 tablespoon lime juice

2 tablespoons olive oil

A pinch of salt and black pepper

1 tablespoon cilantro, chopped

Directions:

In a blender, combine the cream with the scallions, turmeric and the other ingredients except the asparagus and cilantro and pulse well.

Put the sauce in a pan, heat it up over medium heat, add the asparagus and the cilantro, stir, cook for 20 minutes, divide into bowls and serve.

Nutrition: calories 200, fat 12, fiber 2, carbs 5, protein 6

Fennel and Sauce

Preparation time: *10 minutes*

Cooking time: *20 minutes*

Servings: *4*

Ingredients:

2 fennel bulbs, sliced

1 tablespoon avocado oil

2 shallots, chopped

2 garlic cloves, minced

Juice of 1 lime

A pinch of salt and black pepper

2 tablespoons mustard

¼ cup coconut cream

1 tablespoon dill, chopped

Directions:

Heat up a pan with the oil over medium heat, add the shallots and the garlic and sauté for 2 minutes.
Add the mustard and the other ingredients except the fennel, stir and cook for 3 minutes more.
Add the fennel, toss, cook everything for another 15 minutes, divide into bowls and serve.

Nutrition: calories 256, fat 13, fiber 2, carbs 5, protein 6

Baked Sprouts and Tomatoes

Preparation time: *10 minutes*

Cooking time: *25 minutes*

Servings: *4*

Ingredients:

1 pound Brussels sprouts, trimmed and halved

½ pound cherry tomatoes, halved

1 tablespoon avocado oil

4 scallions, chopped

1 teaspoon chili powder

A pinch of salt and black pepper

¼ cup cilantro, chopped

Directions:

In a roasting pan, combine the sprouts with the tomatoes, scallions and the other ingredients, toss and bake at 400 degrees F for 25 minutes.

Divide everything between plates and serve for lunch.

Nutrition: calories 100, fat 3, fiber 1, carbs 2, protein 6

Rosemary Tomatoes and Artichokes

Preparation time: *10 minutes*

Cooking time: *30 minutes*

Servings: *4*

Ingredients:

1 pound tomatoes, halved

2 artichokes, trimmed and halved

1 tablespoon rosemary, chopped

1 tablespoon balsamic vinegar

A pinch of salt and black pepper

2 tablespoons olive oil

1 tablespoon chives, chopped

Directions:

In a roasting pan combine the tomatoes with the artichokes, rosemary and the other ingredients, toss gently and bake at 390 degrees F for 30 minutes. Divide the mix between plates and serve for lunch.

Nutrition: calories 122, fat 12, fiber 1, carbs 3, protein 14

SNACKS

No Bake Golden Energy Bites

Preparation Time: 60 minutes

Cooking Time: 0 minutes

Servings: 6

Ingredients:

1 cup almond butter

¾ cup coconut flakes, unsweetened

6 tablespoons protein powder

1 teaspoon coconut oil

½ teaspoon maple syrup

2 teaspoons turmeric

Directions:

In a bowl, combine all ingredients until a thick dough is formed.

Place dough in a pan lined with parchment paper and spread evenly.

Place in the refrigerator for at least an hour to set.

Remove the bars from the pan and slice to 16 pieces.

Nutrition:

Calories 376, Total Fat 36g, Saturated Fat 5g, Total Carbs 9g, Net Carbs 7g, Protein 6g, Sugar: 5g, Fiber: 2g, Sodium: 194mg, Potassium 310mg

Banana Ginger Bars

Preparation Time: 10 minutes

Cooking Time: 40 minutes

Servings: 5

Ingredients:

2 large ripe bananas, peeled and mashed

1 cup coconut flour

1/3 cup coconut oil

1/3 cup raw honey

6 eggs, pasture-raised

1 tablespoon grated fresh ginger

2 teaspoons cinnamon powder

1 teaspoon ground cardamom powder

1 teaspoon baking soda

2 teaspoons apples cider vinegar

Directions:

Preheat the oven to 350 0F.

Grease a baking dish or line with parchment paper.

In a food processor, combine the bananas, coconut flour, coconut oil, honey, eggs, ginger, cinnamon, and cardamom. Pulse until smooth.

Add the baking soda and apple cider vinegar last and quickly blend.

Pour into the prepared pan.

Bake in the oven for 40 minutes or until a toothpick inserted in the middle comes out clean.

Allow to cool before slicing.

Nutrition:

Calories 364, Total Fat 26g, Saturated Fat 3g, Total Carbs 23g, Net Carbs 22g, Protein 12g, Sugar: 20g, Fiber: 1g, Sodium: 187mg, Potassium 334mg

Kombucha Gummies

Preparation Time: 3 hours

Cooking Time: 10 minutes

Servings: 5

Ingredients:

1 teaspoon grated ginger

1 ½ cups plain kombucha

½ cup grapefruit juice

1 tablespoon grapefruit zest

6 tablespoons honey

1/3 cup gelatin powder

Directions:

Line the bottom of a glass pan with plastic wrap. Set aside.

In a pot, add the ginger and a cup of water. Bring to a boil for 5 minutes. Drain and save the grated ginger.

In another saucepan, combine the kombucha, grapefruit juice, zest, and honey. Sprinkle with the gelatin powder and allow to hydrate for 5 minutes.

Turn on the heat and bring to a boil until the gelatin dissolves. Add in the grated ginger.

Pour into the mixture the prepared glass and chill for 3 hours until the gelatin has set.

Slice into small squares.

Nutrition:
Calories 99, Total Fat 0.03g, Saturated Fat 0g, Total Carbs 26g, Net Carbs 25.9g, Protein 0.4g, Sugar: 26g, Fiber: 0.1g, Sodium: 15mg, Potassium 57mg

Cacao Coffee Protein Bars

Preparation Time: 10 minutes

Cooking Time: 0 minutes

Servings: 6

Ingredients:

2 cups mixed nuts (almond, pecans, cashew and walnuts)

1 cup egg white protein powder

¼ cup cacao powder

3 tablespoons powdered coffee

18 large medjool dates, pitted

¼ cup raw cacao nibs

5 tablespoons water

Directions:

Line a baking pan with parchment paper. Set aside

In a food processor, pulse the nuts, protein powder, cacao powder, and powdered coffee.

Add in the pitted dates and process until fine crumbs form. If dry, add a tablespoon of water until a sticky dough is formed.

Place in a bowl and stir in the cacao nibs.

Transfer the mixture into the pan and spread evenly.

Place inside the fridge and allow to set for 30 minutes before slicing.

Nutrition:

Calories 493, Total Fat 25g, Saturated Fat 3g, Total Carbs 67g, Net Carbs 55g, Protein 12g, Sugar: 50g, Fiber: 12g, Sodium: 2mg, Potassium 956mg

Spicy Taro Crunch

Preparation Time: 10 minutes

Cooking Time: 20 minutes

Servings: 2

Ingredients:

2 cups taro, sliced thinly

1 teaspoon cayenne pepper powder

1 tablespoon olive oil

a pinch of salt

Directions:

Preheat the oven to 3500F.

In a bowl, combine all ingredients. Toss to coat the taro with the spices and seasoning.

Place the taro slices on a baking rack.

Bake for 20 minutes or until the taro becomes crispy.

Nutrition:

Calories 179, Total Fat 7g, Saturated Fat 1g, Total Carbs 28g, Net Carbs 23g, Protein 2g, Sugar: 0.5g, Fiber: 5g, Sodium: 12mg, Potassium 633mg

White Beans Hummus

Preparation Time: 10 minutes

Cooking Time: 5 minutes

Servings: 7

Ingredients:
¼ cup olive oil

1 teaspoon fresh rosemary, chopped

2 cups cooked white beans

¼ cup pure almond butter, unsweetened

1 clove garlic, minced

1 tablespoon lemon juice

¼ cup hot water

¼ teaspoon salt

Directions:

Heat oil in a skillet over medium heat and fry the rosemary for a few minutes. Remove from heat and allow to cool before removing the rosemary leaves. Set aside.

In a food processor, combine the white beans, almond butter, garlic, and lemon juice. Season with salt to taste.

Pulse until smooth. Gradually drizzle with oil and water to adjust the consistency. Save a quarter of the oil.

Place in a bowl and drizzle the remaining olive oil on top.

Serve with vegetable sticks.

Nutrition:

Calories 195, Total Fat 13g, Saturated Fat 2g, Total Carbs 15g, Net Carbs 11g, Protein 7g, Sugar: 0.8g, Fiber: 4g, Sodium: 28mg, Potassium 358mg

Mushroom Pizza

Prep time:10 minutes

Cooking Time:15 minutes

Servings: 4

Ingredients:

2 tablespoons olive oil

¾ pound portobello mushrooms, stems removed

½ cup tomato puree

2 cloves of garlic, minced

½ cup mozzarella cheese, shredded

Salt and pepper to taste

Directions:

Preheat the oven to 350oF.

Brush oil on the inverted side of the mushrooms.

Brush with tomato puree and sprinkle with garlic and mozzarella cheese on top.

Place on a baking pan and bake for 15 minutes.

Nutrition:

Calories 112, Total Fat 7g, Saturated Fat 0.9g, Total Carbs 7g, Net Carbs 5g, Protein 7g, Sugar: 4g, Fiber: 2g, Sodium: 122mg, Potassium 468mg

Quinoa and Beet Kale Dolmades

Preparation Time: 20 minutes

Cooking Time: 50 minutes

Servings: 1

Ingredients:

¼ cup uncooked quinoa

4 leaves dinosaur kale

½ cup beets, grated

1 tablespoons lemon juice

1 teaspoon balsamic vinegar

½ teaspoon orange zest

1 tablespoons olive oil

½ cup water

Instructions

Bring water to a boil over medium flame and cook the quinoa according to package instruction. Drain and allow to cool. Save the warm water.

Place the kale leaves in warm water and blanch for 10 minutes. Set aside and allow water to drain.

In a bowl, combine the quinoa, beets, lemon juice, balsamic vinegar and orange zest.

Place the kale leaves stem side up and add 2 tablespoons of the quinoa mixture. Fold the edges as you would a burrito or spring roll.

Place them in a pan with olive oil and pour ½ cup water.

Cover and bring to a gentle boil over medium low heat. Cook for 45 minutes.

Once the leaves have darkened, remove from the pan and transfer to a plate.

Serve with hummus.

Nutrition:

Calories 490, Total Fat 19g, Saturated Fat 2g, Total Carbs 71g, Net Carbs 55g, Protein 18g, Sugar: 23g, Fiber: 16g, Sodium: 406mg, Potassium 1750mg

Salted Raw Caramel Dip

Preparation Time: minutes

Cooking Time: minutes

Servings: 2

Ingredients:

1 cup soft medjool dates, pitted

1 teaspoon fresh lemon juice

¼ cup almond milk

1 teaspoon vanilla extract

1 tablespoon coconut oil

¼ teaspoon salt

Directions:

Combine all ingredients in a blender or food processor.

Pulse until smooth.

Place in a container and allow to chill before serving.

Nutrition:

Calories 113, Total Fat 7.2g, Saturated Fat 0.01g, Total Carbs 12g, Net Carbs 11.1g, Protein 0.4g, Sugar: 11g, Fiber: 0.9g, Sodium:22 mg, Potassium 112mg

Roasted Red Pepper Hummus with Garlic

Preparation Time: 5 minutes

Cooking Time:0 minutes

Servings: 4

Ingredients:

1 cup chickpea, cooked

2 whole roasted red pepper, seeded and peeled

2 teaspoons minced garlic

4 tablespoons lemon juice

3 tablespoons olive oil

1 teaspoon salt

1 teaspoon black pepper

Directions:

Place all ingredients in a food processor and pulse until smooth.

Place in a bowl and serve with grain-free chips or vegetable chips.

Zucchini and Black Beans Enchiladas

Preparation Time: 10 minutes

Cooking Time: 20 minutes

Servings: 6

Ingredients:

3 large zucchini, diced

3 teaspoons extra virgin olive oil

1 ¼ teaspoon garlic salt

½ small red onion, chopped

1 cup black beans, cooked

¼ cup goat cheese, diced

1 cup tomatoes, diced

A handful of coriander, chopped

salt and pepper to taste

Directions:

Preheat the oven to 3750F.

Place zucchini in a baking tray and drizzle with olive oil. Season with garlic salt.

Bake for 20 minutes or until the edges have browned.

Allow to cool.

Mix all ingredients in a bowl and toss to coat everything.

Serve with vegetable chips.

Nutrition:

Calories 225, Total Fat 9g, Saturated Fat 2g, Total Carbs 22g, Net Carbs 17g, Protein 14g, Sugar: 2g, Fiber: 5g, Sodium: 121mg, Potassium 601mg

Greek Yogurt with Fresh Toppings

Preparation Time: 5 minutes

Cooking Time: 0 minutes

Servings: 1

Ingredients:

1 cup plain Greek yogurt

¼ cup fresh strawberries

1teaspoon organic raw hone

¼ teaspoon cinnamon

Directions:

Combine all ingredients in a bowl.

Chill in the fridge before serving.

Nutrition:

Calories 164, Total Fat 8g, Saturated Fat 1g, Total Carbs 15g, Net Carbs 14g, Protein 9g, Sugar: 14g, Fiber: 1g, Sodium: 150mg, Potassium 348mg

Simple Guacamole

Preparation Time: 5 minutes

Cooking Time: 0 minutes

Servings: 2

Ingredients:

2 tablespoons chopped onion

2 tablespoons chopped cilantro

1 medium chopped avocado

1/8 teaspoon salt

Instructions

Place all ingredients in a food processor.

Pulse until smooth.

Nutrition:

Calories 165, Total Fat 15g, Saturated Fat 2g, Total Carbs 10g, Net Carbs 3g, Protein 2g, Sugar: 1g, Fiber: 7g, Sodium: 8mg, Potassium 507mg

Pumpkin Spiced Apple Chips

Preparation Time: 10 minutes

Cooking Time: 1 hour and 30 minutes

Servings: 3

Ingredients:

2 tablespoons ground cinnamon

1 tablespoons ground ginger

1 ½ teaspoon ground nutmeg

1 ½ teaspoon ground cloves

3 apples, cored and sliced thinly

Directions:

Preheat the oven to 200*0*F.

Line a baking sheet with parchment paper.

In a bowl, toss all ingredients together to coat the apples.

Arrange the seasoned apple slices on the baking sheet.

Place in the oven and bake for 1 ½ hours until the apples are crispy.

Nutrition:
Calories 119, Total Fat 0.9g, Saturated Fat 0.4g, Total Carbs 31g, Net Carbs 23g, Protein 0.9g, Sugar: 19g, Fiber: 8g, Sodium: 3mg, Potassium 244mg

Cranberry Pistachio Energy Bars

Preparation Time: 10 minutes

Cooking Time: 20 minutes

Servings: 5

Ingredients:

1 cup uncooked rolled oat

¾ cup cooked quinoa

¾ cup dried cranberries, chopped

½ cup dry roasted pistachios

1/3 cup unsweetened coconut flakes

2 tablespoons flaxseed meal

1-ounce bittersweet chocolate, chopped

½ cup creamy almond butter

6 tablespoons honey

1 tablespoon olive oil

¼ teaspoon salt

Directions:

Preheat the oven to 350OF.

Spread the oats and quinoa on a baking sheet and bake for 8 minutes until lightly browned.

Place the mixture in a bowl and add in the cranberries, pistachios, coconut flakes, flaxseed, and chocolate.

In a saucepan, combine the almond butter, honey, and olive oil. Mix over low heat for one minute.

Pour the butter mixture into the dry ingredients. Toss to coat.

Press the mixture into a baking dish.

Place the oven and bake for 15 minutes until lightly browned.

Nutrition:

Calories 487, Total Fat 27g, Saturated Fat 4g, Total Carbs 60g, Net Carbs 51g, Protein 13g, Sugar: 33g, Fiber: 9g, Sodium: 135mg, Potassium 550 mg

Orange Mango Gritty with Turmeric and Walnuts

Preparation Time: 5 minutes

Cooking Time: 0 minutes

Servings: 2

Ingredients:

¾ cup plain Greek yogurt

1 cup ice cubes

¾ cup chopped peeled ripe mango

½ cup fresh orange slices

¼ cup chopped toasted walnuts

¼ cup fresh orange juice

1 tablespoon ground flaxseed

2 teaspoons grated fresh turmeric

A dash of grated nutmeg

Directions:

Place all ingredients in a blender and pulse until smooth.

Pour in glasses and serve chilled.

Nutrition:

Calories 245, Total Fat 13g, Saturated Fat 2.3g, Total Carbs 25g, Net Carbs 21g, Protein 11g, Sugar: 19g, Fiber: 4g, Sodium: 91mg, Potassium 731mg

Thai Sesame Edamame

Preparation Time: 10 minutes

Cooking Time:1 hour and 10 minutes

Servings: 6

Ingredients:

4 cups edamame pods

1 tablespoon dark sesame oil

1 tablespoon rice vinegar

1 teaspoon toasted sesame seeds

3 tablespoons water

½ teaspoon salt

½ teaspoon ground black pepper

Directions:

Preheat the oven to 300ºF.

Line a baking sheet with aluminum foil. Set aside.

Place all ingredients in a bowl and toss to coat the edamame pods with the seasoning.

Arrange the seasoned edamame pods in the baking sheet.

Bake for 1 hour and 10 minutes until the pods are crispy.

Nutrition:

Calories 149, Total Fat 8g, Saturated Fat 0.9g, Total Carbs 10g, Net Carbs 5g, Protein 11g, Sugar: 2g, Fiber: 5g, Sodium:9 mg, Potassium 454mg

Sweet Potato Keto Muffins

Preparation Time: 15 minutes

Cooking Time: 35 minutes

Servings: 6

Ingredients:

1 small sweet potato, cooked

1 egg, pasture-raised

¾ cup coconut milk

2 tablespoons olive oil

½ cup pure maple syrup

1 cup brown rice flour

¼ cup coconut flour

1 tablespoon baking powder

1 tablespoon ground cinnamon

1 teaspoon ground ginger

1 teaspoon ground turmeric

1/8 teaspoon ground cloves

1/8 teaspoon ground nutmeg

½ teaspoon salt

Directions:

Preheat the oven to 400OF.

Peel the cooked potato and place in a bowl. Mash gently with fork or masher.

Add in the eggs, coconut milk, olive oil, and maple syrup. Mix until well combined.

In a separate bowl, mix the rice flour, coconut flour, baking powder, cinnamon, ginger, turmeric, cloves, and nutmeg.

Gradually add the milk mixture into the flour mixture. Fold until well-combined.

Grease muffin cups then pour batter into the pan until ¾ full.

Bake in the oven for 35 minutes.

Nutrition:

Calories 311, Total Fat 14g, Saturated Fat 2g, Total Carbs 43g, Net Carbs 40g, Protein 5g, Sugar: 18g, Fiber: 3g, Sodium: 41mg, Potassium 329mg

Beet Chips

Preparation Time: 10 minutes

Cooking Time: 1 hour and 30 minutes

Servings: 2

Ingredients:

3 medium beets, peeled and sliced thinly

1 tablespoon olive oil

Salt to taste

Directions:

Preheat the oven to 350*0*F.

Place all ingredients in a bowl and toss to coat.

Arrange the seasoned beet slices on a baking tray lined with aluminum foil.

Bake in the oven for 1 hour and 30 minutes.

Make sure to flip the beets halfway through the cooking time.

Nutrition:
Calories 120, Total Fat 7g, Saturated Fat 1g, Total Carbs 12g, Net Carbs 9g, Protein 2g, Sugar: 8g, Fiber: 3g, Sodium: 210mg, Potassium 921mg

Conclusion

Thank you for reading through to the end of this book, *Intermittent Fasting 16/8*!

The next step is to determine what you want your intermittent 16/8 fasting cycle to be. Then go out and fill your pantry with clean, whole foods that will benefit your body with intermittent fasting or by following the Ketogenic Diet alongside your intermittent fasting lifestyle!

You should have the preliminary information you need to get started with making your own snacks and meals to maximize your weight loss potential and limit your carbohydrates and fat store accumulation.

Get ready to feel the health benefits and the amazing changes in your body as you utilize a 16/8 intermittent fasting plan. Shed weight and belly fat quickly and improve your overall health as well as reduce your risk for certain diseases long term.

There are plenty of other sources of information about intermittent fasting and the ketogenic diet. Thank you for choosing this book and using it as your guide to getting started! There is always more to learn and always more information, but the chapters are written hear should offer you the basics for getting started and put to rest any concerns you may have had.